Listening for What Matters

ADVANCED PRAISE FOR *LISTENING FOR WHAT MATTERS*

"The concept of patient-centered medical care, originally a call for clinicians to attend to the patients' psychosocial as well as biomedical needs particular to each patient, has since been co-opted as a marketing tool by the commercial enterprise that is American medicine. A 'patient-centered' practice now boasts evening hours and a good web site—but may or may not be attentive to the issues so critical to clinical practice that Weiner and Schwartz explore here. Their work on contextualized care reclaims this territory and redefines what it means to be patient-centered, with a robust and pragmatic model useful in teaching, practice, and in further research on physician behavior."

Raymond Curry, MD, FACP
Senior Associate Dean for Educational Affairs, University of Illinois College of Medicine
Charter Member, American Academy on Communication in Health Care

"Weiner and Schwartz take you behind the scenes in failed and successful patient/doctor interactions, as well as clinical trials and medical education classrooms. In the process, they illuminate the reasons for successful and unsuccessful patient/doctor interactions. This is a book that should be read by all patients who want to get the most from their interactions with their physicians. This is a book that should be read by all medical students, physicians, health care executives, and policy workers. There is something for everyone. This is a highly readable exploration of the patient/doctor relationship and how all involved parties can improve it."

Walter J. McDonald MD, MACP
Emeritus CEO American College of Physicians

"This book should be required reading for anyone teaching medical students and residents. This groundbreaking book has the potential to incite a revolution in graduate medical education. The writers have scientifically demonstrated that many physicians are not skilled at interviewing patients with complex medical and well as psychosocial issues. We ignore the information shared in this valuable book at our own peril."

Michael R. Wasserman, MD
Director, Nursing Home QIN-QIO, Health Services Advisory Group, Inc.

"This fascinating story summarizes decades of research by its authors, Dr. Saul J. Weiner and Dr. Alan Schwartz, into the importance of the 'patient's context' in prescribing care. Physicians who apply guidelines based on biomedical criteria without modification to fit the situational, demographic, cultural, and social dimensions of the individual patient are at risk of a serious medical error: prescribing 'the right treatment' to the 'wrong patient.' The book makes an important contribution to an understanding of the requirements for patient-centered care, one that emphasizes the importance of physician as well as patient engagement in diagnosing context and sorting out the treatments that the individual patient wants and needs."

John E. Wennberg, MD, MPH
Peggy Y. Thomson Professor Emeritus, Evaluative Clinical Sciences &Founder
Director Emeritus of The Dartmouth Institute for Health Policy and Clinical Practice

Listening for What Matters

Avoiding Contextual Errors in Health Care

STAFF PHYSICIAN, JESSE BROWN VA MEDICAL CENTER
DEPUTY DIRECTOR, VA CENTER FOR INNOVATION
IN COMPLEX CHRONIC HEALTHCARE
PROFESSOR OF MEDICINE, PEDIATRICS AND MEDICAL EDUCATION
UNIVERSITY OF ILLINOIS AT CHICAGO

ALAN SCHWARTZ
THE MICHAEL REESE ENDOWED PROFESSOR
OF MEDICAL EDUCATION,
DEPARTMENT OF MEDICAL EDUCATION
RESEARCH PROFESSOR, DEPARTMENT OF PEDIATRICS
UNIVERSITY OF ILLINOIS AT CHICAGO

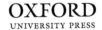

OXFORD
UNIVERSITY PRESS

OXFORD

UNIVERSITY PRESS

Oxford University Press is a department of the University of
Oxford. It furthers the University's objective of excellence in research,
scholarship, and education by publishing worldwide.

Oxford   New York
Auckland   Cape Town   Dar es Salaam   Hong Kong   Karachi
Kuala Lumpur   Madrid   Melbourne   Mexico City   Nairobi
New Delhi   Shanghai   Taipei   Toronto

With offices in
Argentina   Austria   Brazil   Chile   Czech Republic   France   Greece
Guatemala   Hungary   Italy   Japan   Poland   Portugal   Singapore
South Korea   Switzerland   Thailand   Turkey   Ukraine   Vietnam

Oxford is a registered trademark of Oxford University Press
in the UK and certain other countries.

Published in the United States of America by
Oxford University Press
198 Madison Avenue, New York, NY 10016

Library of Congress Cataloging-in-Publication Data
Weiner, Saul J., author.
Listening for what matters : avoiding contextual errors in health care / by Saul J. Weiner,
Alan Schwartz.
    p. ; cm.
Includes bibliographical references and index.
ISBN 978-0-19-022899-6 (alk. paper)
I. Schwartz, Alan, 1970–, author.   II. Title.
[DNLM: 1. Communication.   2. Physician–Patient Relations.   3. Attitude of Health Personnel.
4. Medical Errors—prevention & control. W 62]
R729.8
610.289—dc23
2015020732

CONTENTS

FOREWORD   VII

ACKNOWLEDGMENTS   XI

INTRODUCTION   XIII

PART I **The Problem**

  1. Observing the Problem   3

  2. Measuring the Problem   25

  3. The Problem Is Everywhere   58

  4. What We Hear that Physicians Don't   76

PART II **Solutions**

  5. Causes   95

  6. Better Teaching, Better Doctors   120

  7. Is Lasting Change Possible?   137

  8. What We Can't Measure that Matters   165

  9. Bringing Context Back into Care   186

NOTES   199

BIBLIOGRAPHY   203

INDEX   207

In the nostalgic days of Norman Rockwell, general practitioners practiced in small-to-medium-sized communities and had lifelong relationships with their patients. Some of these relationships and this knowledge base persist among primary care providers today, particularly those who have looked after their patients for many years. However, for many more patients, health care is fragmented, with multiple providers and short periods of direct physician interaction. Patients' lives are increasingly complex, as many change jobs and move frequently. In the 2008 "Great Recession," we witnessed the way in which well-established individuals at various social class levels became unemployed.

What happens when doctors no longer understand how their patients' lives affect their health care? In their research into "contextualizing care," Saul Weiner and Alan Schwartz have tried to understand how and why physicians fail to incorporate patient context in care planning and how to more effectively deal with these failures. These contextual errors are medical errors—"failure of a planned action to be completed as intended or the use of the wrong plan to achieve an aim"—and Schwartz and Weiner's studies demonstrate that they are widespread.

In tackling their challenge, they have created novel investigative and educational methodologies and have provided additional insights into the way in which physicians generally communicate with patients. Ten broad domains of patient context are identified, including access to care, social support, competing responsibilities, financial situation, relationship with healthcare providers, skills and abilities, emotional state, cultural/spiritual beliefs, environment, and attitudes toward illness.

Weiner and Schwartz have focused their attention upon the most efficient and effective way for the busy physician to understand the context of the patient's life, so as to help with a sensible and workable plan. Clearly, in a 15-minute interaction, the physician cannot glean information in all of the relevant domains identified by the authors. Rather, the authors focus on the physician's ability to identify "red flags," which suggest the need for further probing to understand the context of the patient's life. The "red flags" may be in the form of statements made by the patients or communicated through the patient's behavior; for example, frequently missing appointments. With physician and institutional review board (IRB) approval, they audiotaped the interactions between "standardized patients" (actors playing patients) and real patients with physicians. In analyzing the tapes, they developed a coding system called "4C" to identify the outcomes of each encounter—Content Coding for Contextualization of Care. Their coding asks the questions: "Does the patient demonstrate a possible contextual factor that may be a red flag? If there is a red flag, does the physician ask about it? If the patient revealed a contextual factor, was it in response to a probe by the physician? If there is a contextual factor, did the physician address it in the care plan?"

Although often a useful record for evaluating care, the patient chart is not a reliable source for identifying failures to deal with patient context. The authors provide thoughtful and interesting approaches to the use of audio tapes to record physician/patient interactions using standardized patients in experimental models and actual patients in quality-improvement efforts. The studies indicate that a significant portion of care plans are flawed because they do not adequately address patient context, even when "red flags" are raised by the patient's comments or behavior. Controlled studies of learning by medical students indicated that they can learn how to identify aspects of patient context and take these into consideration in caring for the patient. Aggressive efforts to educate residents and practitioners showed that their awareness of patient context can be improved and health plans modified to reflect this context. However, it is as yet unclear what the longevity of the learned behaviors may be.

Audio studies are complex operationally, technically, and ethically. As the authors point out, in many other industries, recordings are made in order to assess quality, but this technique is a relatively new and infrequently applied strategy in medicine. Their recordings yielded information about a broad spectrum of physician communication skills and strategies which, at times, were appalling. Frequent interruption of the patient, failure to hear what the patient is saying, use of a rote checklist to obtain a history, a complete failure to understand why the patient has come to see the physician and how the patient perceives his or her problem, are only a few of the weaknesses these studies revealed.

Although some of these studies were conducted in the offices of private practice physicians, many were conducted within VA administration hospitals. The special issues confronted by VA patients and the structure of the provider workforce in the VA, raises questions about generalizability of the research findings in this population. However, the work is extremely useful in identifying methodologies, with appropriate modifications, which may be important in improving education and performance during a wide variety of patient–doctor interactions.

To what extent is the concept of contextualizing care in and of itself an important notion? Currently, there is widespread commitment to the concept of patient-centered care, that is, care that is respectful and responsive to individual patient preferences, needs, and values. Don Berwick has defined patient-centered care as, "The experience (to the extent the informed, individual patient desires it) of transparency, individualization, recognition, respect, dignity and choice in all matters without exception, related to one's personal circumstances in relationships in healthcare." These definitions emphasize the importance of contextualizing care as described by Weiner and Schwartz.

If completely implemented, patient-centered care would include all of the considerations of contextual care. However, the concept of patient-centered care is so broad that methods to evaluate it require attention to specific aspects. Contextualizing care provides just such an opportunity and allows application across the broad range of domains identified by the authors. At the same time, it has offered opportunities to develop methodologies that could be applied much more widely. The detailed description of how the authors undertake their investigations and deal with the ethical and bureaucratic issues associated with audiotaping of patient-doctor exchanges are important contributions to understanding how to improve care in a manner that does not ordinarily reveal itself in the medical records.

Another important contribution from these studies is the understanding that addressing some aspects of patient-centered care need not dramatically increase the amount of time required by the patient–doctor interaction. The studies also highlight the challenges associated with bringing other health professionals into the process of patient-centered care.

As these methodologies are refined, one can hope that they will be applied more broadly in other parts of the healthcare delivery system, both as parts of investigations and as continuous quality improvement. Medical educators have been writing and working extensively on methods to improve communication skills for students at every level of their career. The results of the studies reported in this book indicate that much needs to be done if the patient–doctor interaction can live up to its expectations across the healthcare system. The methods proposed by the authors offer some real opportunities to accomplish this goal. Their explicit identification of the context of the patient's situation is a central part of the patient–physician interaction. The subsequent plan for the patient and physician arising from the context is an important contribution. The authors' experience with audiotaping and analyzing the recorded interaction opens important new avenues toward improving the quality of health care.

Kenneth Shine, MD
Past President, Institute of Medicine of
the National Academies

ACKNOWLEDGMENTS

The research we review in this book is the product of a decade of work with many outstanding people. We are particularly indebted to our research team and collaborators. They play keys roles in many chapters, but their intelligence, diligence, and creativity goes well beyond what we have been able to capture here.

We commend the medical students, residents, clinical staff, and physicians who have participated in our research and quality improvement projects at University of Illinois Chicago (UIC), in the Veterans Health Administration (VA) system, and around the Midwest. These dedicated professionals not only agreed to allow themselves to be observed and recorded doing their work, but in most cases welcomed it as part of their goal to continually improve the care and health of their patients. We are heartened by their trust and commitment. This work also would be impossible without the help of our standardized patient actors and of real patients, particularly veterans, who have carried concealed audio-recorders into their visits. The research was supported by the Department of Veterans Affairs, Veterans Health Administration, Office of Research and Development, Health Services Research & Development. Funds for the quality improvement project are from the Veterans Integrated Service Network (VISN) 12. The views expressed in this book do not necessarily reflect the position or policy of the Department of Veterans Affairs or the United States government. Portions of the research also were funded by a National Board of Medical Examiners® (NBME®) Edward J. Stemmler, MD Medical Education Research Fund grant. The project does not necessarily reflect NBME policy, and NBME support provides no official endorsement.

Simon Auster has been an extraordinary source of insight and guidance from the inception of this work up to the present. Amy Binns-Calvey provided valuable feedback on nearly every chapter, for which we are extremely grateful. Craig Panner, our editor at Oxford University Press, was very helpful in shaping the book and helping us work through how best to tell these stories. Of course, any errors or omissions are ours alone.

We consider this some of our most important work, and we have been supported throughout by some profoundly important people: Suzanne Griffel, Karen Weiner, M. G. Bertulfo, and Ari Schwartz. No words of thanks would be enough.

SJW & AS
Chicago, April 2015

Getting sick and needing health care are part of life for nearly all of us. When serious health problems strike they can be profoundly disruptive to our usual routines, and when they linger they force us into new behaviors. When this happens we discover how our health and health needs are inextricably connected to every aspect of our lives. If we used to feel confident, we may now feel unsure in ways that disrupt well-honed coping strategies developed during a healthier time. If we used to feel strong, we may now feel vulnerable and frail. At a more practical level, simply fitting in the doctor's appointments, the bandage changes, the medication refills, and adjustments to accommodate physical symptoms often involve trade-offs as our lives have to "give" somewhere.

As obvious as this all seems to anyone coping with health issues, healthcare experts are prone to overlooking the obvious. How can that be? Doctors care for the sick day in and day out, seeing in countless ways how people look and function when they are ill, and using the best available science to manage their care.

Do visits to the doctor seem impersonal? Are doctors uninterested in us as people? When doctors are rude or indifferent, is it simply unpleasant, or does it worsen the quality of the care we receive and, ultimately, our health?

Many doctors clearly care. They are empathic, treat us warmly, give us ample time, address our concerns, and make themselves readily accessible. When you are feeling vulnerable and uncertain, such support is welcome. But does it really matter? What are the health implications of having a nice doctor?

The proposition of this book is that although how healthcare providers communicate is intrinsically important to us as patients—we all appreciate doctors who seem caring—hidden and unmeasured skills distinguish providers who grasp the connections between our health needs and our unique life circumstances from those who are merely genial. The former help us find ways to cope and function as well as we possibly can under those circumstances. We call that process "contextualizing care."

These are a practical set of skills. When a doctor has them and uses them, patients walk out of the office feeling as though they have plans that make sense for *them*. These plans accommodate the obstacle course of their lives, including the anxieties and feelings evoked by illness as well as more mundane challenges, like not having a car to get to a lab regularly for blood tests before work. On the other hand, when doctors lack these skills, patients walk out unsure. They may be hopeful because the doctors seemed positive and nice, but the plans do not quite fit the puzzles that are their lives.

Most health care does not happen in the healthcare setting. Much of it does not even involve doctors or nurses. It happens at home, or at work or on vacation as millions of people try to keep track of their pills, or cope with side effects, or travel to and from medical appointments, or turn to family and friends, or the Internet for advice and help. To be effective, healthcare providers have to understand and incorporate their patients' complicated lives. These are skills and ways of thinking, not merely sentiments. They demand an approach to supporting patients that begins with an appreciation of how the circumstances of those lives relate to their care.

We understand the clinical interaction as one individual simply trying to be helpful to another. The person who is helping has a toolkit, which is her or his medical training. The person seeking help has a healthcare need. The one with the toolkit—the medical training—may or may not need it, and he or she may need to reach beyond it. As a colleague of ours once put it: The helpful doctor is prepared to stand on his or her head if that is what will help the patient.

Much of the writing about quality of health care falls broadly into two categories. In the first is the extensive interest in improving the science and safety of how care is delivered. Thousands of studies, reports, and books detail and emphasize the importance of what has been called "evidence-based medicine" as it applies to the individual patient, or systems approaches to care that minimize the risks of medical error in large healthcare organizations. In the second category are books and medical school courses that focus on "humanistic medicine" or "doctoring," which emphasize empathy and good communication behavior.

We wrote this book to chart a new direction, incorporating something from each of these two major categories. On the surface, our interest seems to fall into the humanistic camp. We will talk a lot about the importance of being good listeners, of engaging, and of caring. Dig deeper and you will see these qualities are secondary to our true interest. Our focus is on whether those in the healthcare system who interact with patients understand that their role is entirely to help patients solve healthcare problems, and whether they have learned how to do that effectively when faced with uniquely individual patients.

Is this really new? After all, the Institute of Medicine of the National Academy of Sciences defined "patient-centered care" years ago as "providing care that is respectful of and responsive to individual patient preferences, needs, and values, and ensuring that patient values guide all clinical decisions." That is a good definition, but how does one do it? How does one know whether and when it is happening? How is it measured? How do we make someone better at it?

When it comes to science and safety, physicians are tracked using a growing number of "performance measures." These are metrics based on hundreds of guidelines that are, in turn, assembled from research studies that compare various forms of treatment. But the guidelines are called "guidelines" (rather than, say, "directives") because they are not assumed to be appropriate or even feasible in all situations. How can we tell whether physicians are adapting guidelines when the recommended care will not help—or may even harm—a particular patient, due to that patient's life context?

In all fairness, it is both important and much simpler to evaluate whether healthcare professionals are following guidelines than whether they are contextualizing care. After all, once there is a guideline, all one has to do is check whether physicians are following it. Evidence of adherence to guidelines can be extracted either from the medical record or from the claims data that go to insurers, based on whether the right tests were ordered or treatments recommended based on the recorded diagnosis. In contrast, there is no checklist for whether care is personalized. Assessing whether care is appropriate for a particular patient's life situation depends on having information that is only disclosed in the intimacy of the physician–patient encounter and rarely recorded in the chart. Thus, patient-centered care is valued, but rarely evaluated.

We have attempted to integrate the sentiments of humanistic care—the uniqueness of the individual—with the science of measurement, which is typically applied to groups of individuals that for the purposes of analyses are considered similar. Why is it so important to measure attention to individual context in care planning? We invoke here Osborne and Gaebler's often quoted dictum:

What gets measured gets done
If you don't measure results, you can't tell success from failure
If you can't see success, you can't reward it
If you can't reward success, you're probably rewarding failure
If you can't see success, you can't learn from it
If you can't recognize failure, you can't correct it
If you can demonstrate results, you can win public support[1]

If we do not assess whether care is contextual, but assiduously track whether guidelines are followed, then we promote a mechanized approach to care that neglects individual needs.

At the same time, we are hesitant to call our approach "doctoring" or the "art of medicine." These terms are unassailably positive, but also too vague; the "good" doctor who is "humanistic" and practices the "art of medicine" evokes a Norman Rockwell sentiment rather than learnable skills for being helpful in the clinical context. Moreover, "doctoring" suggests that these skills belong only to physicians, whereas we have come to appreciate that everyone in the health system who interacts with patients needs to consider the patients' circumstances when assisting or supporting them. Hence, there is a role for "doctoring" at the front desk when a patient who has previously always been on time starts showing up late repeatedly and looks flustered: "Mr. Davis," the front desk clerk might ask, "You look like you've been having a hard time getting here lately, and that it's been tough for you. Is everything okay?" Contrast that with "Mr. Davis, since you're more than 20 minutes late I'm going to have to reschedule you." Which one looks like "doctoring"?

Thus, we have adopted a technically precise but distinctly unsentimental term: "contextualizing care." This book is fundamentally about the contextual thinking skills that separate a professional healthcare worker from a technician or robot. Without them, a doctor is not doctoring and a clerk is just a clerk.

This book follows the path of our exploration into contextual thinking in health care. The first four chapters, under the heading Part I, "The Problem," describe what we know about how physicians succeed or fail at contextual thinking with patients, and how we know it. Chapter 1, titled "Observing the Problem," is structured around a series of case examples that illustrate what happens when clinicians overlook patient context, and how care planning changes when they finally take it into account. One of the goals of this first chapter is to assure that readers understand what this book is about and why it matters. We also propose some hypotheses about why failures to incorporate patient context into care planning occur—both because of assumptions healthcare providers tend to make about patients' lives and circumstances and because of a simple tendency not to think about their lives and circumstances at all. Finally, we consider what it might take to think contextually—which essentially involves asking patients questions and knowing what questions to ask. We conclude with an illustration of why thinking contextually is not a linear "checklist" process. At its best, it emerges out of an engaged interaction between two individuals, one in the healing role and the other seeking health through health care. "Engagement" is an important concept that describes a particular kind of interaction between individuals, and we devote some time to it later in the book.

The second chapter, "Measuring the Problem," transitions from anecdotes and hypotheses to systematic inquiry, detailing our early research. We begin by describing some of the big ideas that have impacted health-care delivery in the last few decades—the evidence-based medicine movement, the development of clinical practice guidelines, and attention to medical error. Laypersons may not be aware of the extent to which a bandwagon or two comes along every 15 years and dominates discourse in health care. Bandwagons are noisy; they tend to drown everything else out. In Chapter 2, we discuss how the emphasis on standardizing care could draw attention away from the importance of adapting care to individual patients' differences, and how the emphasis on the medical record prevents us from seeing mistakes made during the visit that never make it into the chart.

With this as a backdrop, we describe the conundrum we found ourselves in, trying to study a problem that leaves no footprint in the medical record. After considering several options, we realized we had to observe physician decision-making directly by sending "secret shopper" patients undercover into doctors' practices to portray cases that challenge physicians to think contextually. This, in turn, posed a considerable logistical challenge, which included winning the trust of a large group of physicians in order for them to agree to be "subjects" in such a venture, manipulating the medical record to create fake patient medical charts, and training actors to do what they came to call "the con," whereby they adopt the personae of real patients while adhering to a script to get a specific job done. The success of this work depended on the courage of the doctors who participated and on several high-level administrators in the Veterans Health Administration system—where we collected much of our data—who took steps to protect us from larger forces that wanted to shut us down. Finally, we review the fruits of this labor: the evidence that even when actors drop huge hints that there are life factors interfering with their care, doctors tend to miss these, instead, sending patients out the door with plans that look great on paper but make no sense for the patient.

Having documented that physicians overlook context more often than not, even when we were sure that context mattered to care planning, our next step was to see how often context matters in actual practice. To do that, we had to transition from employing actors with contrived problems, each customized to test clinician attention to context, to recruiting real patients with real problems and asking them to carry the hidden audio-recorders. Chapter 3 describes this phase of our work. What we stood to gain was insight about how often effective care really hinges on a personalized approach in which individual life circumstances are a key factor in planning. We also were interested in seeing whether the poor performance we observed when clinicians interacted with actors was, in fact, representative of care real patients receive in practice. Our title for Chapter 3, "The Problem is Everywhere," hints at what we found.

The cost of going from fake to real patients was losing the simplicity and precision of measuring and comparing clinicians' performance based on challenges that we had embedded in cases. With real patients, there is no way to know what, if anything, will come up during a visit—what vital information regarding life situations and potential obstacles to effective care will emerge. Hence, we had to develop a flexible and reliable system for assessing the clinician's attention to contextual information when we would not know the context in advance. Finally, because we were going to study real patient interactions, we had a unique opportunity to compare healthcare outcomes of patients whose care is contextualized with those whose care plans are inattentive to their life needs and circumstances.

As with our strategy of introducing fake patients into the clinical setting, enlisting real patients to carry concealed audio recorders into their visits poses a set of challenges we had to address. Whereas others have employed unannounced standardized patients in the clinical setting, as far as we are aware asking real patients to covertly record their encounters was a first. We discuss how we addressed the ethical and legal issues as well as the potential concerns of participants, clinicians and patients alike.

Chapter 4, "What We Hear that Physicians Don't," is a bit of a technical dive into how our research team works with the data collected from audio-recorded encounters. In particular, we introduce the coding system we developed, called "Content Coding for Contextualization of Care," or "4C." By coding content, in contrast to coding of process, 4C requires following the thread and logic of a conversation. In this chapter we also discuss why we had to develop 4C, namely, because other approaches to assessing communication that are commonly employed in doctor–patient communication research do not capture information on whether clinicians are actually paying attention to and addressing key information that comes up during the encounter.

Part II, titled "Solutions," comprising the remaining chapters, takes stock of what we have learned about the challenges of contextualizing care, and how we can use that knowledge both to reduce contextual errors and to empower patients to ensure they receive care that is not only based on clinical evidence but adapted to their needs and circumstances. We begin with "Causes," in which we ask, essentially, "How does context get overlooked?" Although they were not designed to answer the "Why?" question, after studying thousands of encounters, we have identified six attributes that lead a physician to overlook context, or to appreciate and incorporate it, and Chapter 5 is where we share them.

Chapter 6, "Better Teaching, Better Doctors," describes an educational program we developed and assessed, using a research method most commonly associated with the study of clinical interventions—the randomized controlled trial. We sought to discover whether a brief experiential curriculum could prepare physicians to be more effective at contextualizing care, as measured by actors role-playing standardized patients in a performance laboratory. We worked with fourth-year medical school students for this project because they seemed at the right point in the developmental trajectory of a physician—not too junior to appreciate the complexities of patient care, but not so far along as to be irrevocably fixed in their ways. Although the results of this study were gratifying—we saw improvement—subsequent work with more rigorous measures proved that changing physician behavior is a bigger challenge. This becomes evident in a second study we describe, conducted with more sophisticated measurement, in which clinicians were evaluated with both standardized patients in the lab and unannounced standardized patients in the actual practice setting. What physicians were able to show they could do (i.e., their skills) turned out not to be the same as what they actually do in practice (i.e., their performance). We talk about this distinction here.

One of the lessons of Chapter 6 is that one cannot transform with a mini-course how physicians think about and approach their work. Real change likely requires frequent assessment with feedback, based on what is observed in actual practice. Furthermore, altering something as complex as behavioral interaction requires frequent reinforcement. We concluded that to make all this happen we would need to enlist actual patients willing to routinely audio record their encounters, or employ unannounced standardized patients, or some combination thereof. We would have to find a way to continuously provide feedback with analyzed data from the audio to clinicians, along with easy-to-understand information about their performance. And, finally, we would have to do this in a way that would not alienate doctors but engage them so that they saw the process as an opportunity to learn. Hence, Chapter 7, "Is Lasting Change Possible?" describes such a project undertaken at two large outpatient clinics at VA medical centers in Chicago. Although we began with a focus exclusively on physicians, the project expanded to include clerical staff, nurses, and clinical pharmacists. Chapter 7 describes how we provide everyone on the care team with data on a recurring basis for self and group reflection that illustrates the value of contextualizing care. Repeatedly seeing one's own lapses in the work that one prides oneself at doing well—combined with the reward of seeing improvement with effort—is the most compelling driver of change.

Chapter 8, "What We Can't Measure that Matters," is about the variations in how clinicians attend to context that we are not assessing. Why do we discuss this? First, we want to be transparent about what we consider the limitations of our work. We think we are better at identifying which providers are performing poorly than at discriminating among those who are doing well. Second, we have conceptualized the elements of a healing interaction that comprehensively attend to context, so this chapter may be regarded as scaffolding for the structure that lies atop our foundation. We are indebted to our colleague, Simon Auster, for his decades of reflection on the topics discussed, including engagement and boundary clarity. Finally, we connect the dots here between the work we have done thus far and what lies ahead.

Chapter 9, "Bringing Context Back into Care," distills what we have learned and what is left to do not only for physicians, but for hospitals, payers, regulators, medical educators, and patients. This chapter encapsulates both our hopes and our frustrations with efforts to instill patient-centered care.

If you choose to read this book from cover to cover we hope you will experience some of the surprise and discovery we have experienced along the way. One of the challenges we faced in writing this book as two authors, at a practical level, is narrative voice. For over a decade we have collaborated closely on this work, bringing different skills and fulfilling complementary roles. Perhaps the most natural way of telling the story would have been to imagine that the two of us were sitting around an open fire with you, the reader. Each of us would take turns, referring to the other by name when relating anecdotes. We might alternate from Alan telling how " . . . Saul went out to meet with a group of physicians in a small suburb to see if we could send them fake patients . . ." to Saul explaining that " . . . Alan suggested we e-mail physicians to see whether they could tell us which of their patients was fake . . . ." Although this style works well around a campfire, our editor convinced us that it is not a good way to talk to an audience from the pages of a book. Hence, throughout, we have adopted the third person plural, "we." In fact, it is often just one of us to whom we are referring. If it sounds like something a doctor would do, it is probably Saul. If it sounds like something a research methodologist would do, it is probably Alan. If it sounds like something that neither could do alone, it probably was both.

Finally, a comment about names and identifiers. We have changed the names of all clinicians, staff, and patients. We have only retained the names of individuals whose identities and titles were significant to the narrative and who agreed to be named.

PART I

The Problem

Observing the Problem

"A technician can be defined as one who knows every aspect of his job–except its ultimate purpose and social consequences."
—SIR RICHARD W. LIVINGSTON (ATTRIB.)

INTRODUCING CONTEXT: WHAT IS MISSING FROM BIOMEDICALLY FOCUSED CARE?

Amelia Garcia is a reserved, patient, and polite 46-year-old woman with kidney failure from diabetes who speaks limited English. She had returned repeatedly to the emergency room (ER)—four times in the last year—at the University of Illinois hospital on the west side of Chicago (UIC) because she had missed her hemodialysis appointments. Despite her kidney problems, she appeared quite well when she arrived at the ER for the fifth time. Because of the missed dialysis sessions, however, her serum potassium level was dangerously high, putting her at significant risk for an unstable heart rhythm that could be deadly. Each time she showed up in the emergency room, doctors would select a therapy based on the results of her blood tests and electrocardiogram (ECG). On this occasion, when her serum potassium level was nearly 7.0, a life-threatening level, her ECG showed peaked t-waves and, more ominously, early widening of the QRS complex, a warning of heart trouble. As on each of her visits, the

ER staff inserted an IV into her arm. To manage her high potassium, she was treated initially with calcium gluconate, which immediately stabilizes the heart muscle to reduce the chance of a fatal rhythm disturbance. After being stabilized, she was transferred to the nephrology unit for hemodialysis. As on prior admissions, the plan was to send her home later that day or the following morning, her emergency managed, with reminders not to miss her dialysis again and a warning that doing so could be fatal. ER staff refer to patients like Ms. Garcia who turn up repeatedly as "frequent flyers." In her medical record, she also was described as "hemodialysis noncompliant" at each previous visit.

But this visit was different. Before she was discharged, a medical student caring for her asked her why she missed her dialysis. Although the student did not speak Spanish, there was a Spanish bilingual medical student on the team, who translated. Ms. Garcia explained that she lived in a three bedroom house with her seven children, plus her daughter's husband and their new baby. One son, age 15, had received a kidney transplant and was being cared for by a pediatric nephrologist at UIC. Another son, age 17, has cerebral palsy and also received his care at UIC. Ms. Garcia described her home environment as a happy one and said they manage financially on her disability insurance, her sons' disability insurance, and her son-in-law's paycheck.

Ms. Garcia explained that she is dialyzed at a site that is not only far from her home but also far from UIC. She comes to UIC virtually weekly because of her sons' medical needs, which sometimes conflict with her dialysis schedule. The transportation service to and from the hemodialysis center, which is located on the far south side of Chicago, is not reliable, and the staff there have not been helpful when she has discussed her transportation needs with them. The service will only pick her up at her home and take her to and from dialysis—there is no way for her to get directly from the dialysis center to UIC or back.

When the inpatient team raised with her the possibility of moving her hemodialysis over to UIC, Ms. Garcia responded enthusiastically. She had not been aware she could get long-term dialysis at the hospital. She commented that she could then bring her son to his nephrology appointment on the same days she came for hemodialysis. That would solve her transportation problem and enable her to get the prescribed three times weekly hemodialysis. The medical team contacted the social worker who managed hemodialysis and she facilitated the transfer of care. A review of Ms. Garcia's medical record almost a year later showed no subsequent ER visits or hospital admissions.

INATTENTION TO CONTEXT: DOCTORS WITH BLINDERS

This book is about the failure of the medical profession to recognize the relevance of a patient's life context to planning and implementing effective care. In particular, it is about doctors failing to ask their patients fundamental questions. Reflecting on how doctors approached Ms. Garcia, two major themes emerge: First, they were inquisitive and responsive to the biomedical aspects of her care. They knew that bad things can happen inside the body when patients miss their hemodialysis, and held themselves accountable for finding out what they were. This process involved asking relevant questions such as, "What metabolic abnormalities should I consider in this patient?" They sought and found the answers, then intervened promptly to correct those that were life-threatening. Second, they evidenced a distinct lack of curiosity about the basis for the behaviors that led to the failure in her care—what we have identified as the contextual aspects of her care—namely, why she kept missing her hemodialysis in the first place. They were aware enough of the problem to give it a label—"noncompliant"—and to admonish her not to miss her hemodialysis anymore, but the spirit of inquiry or ownership of the situation that would be manifest if her physicians felt responsible for engaging Ms. Garcia as a person, rather than as a physiological specimen, was missing. In short, they did not wonder about *why* Ms. Garcia, who evidenced no other self-destructive behaviors, would repeatedly return to the unappealing environment of a crowded urban emergency room with a self-inflicted life-threatening condition. They repeatedly failed to ask the right question: "Ms. Garcia, can you please tell us why you keep missing your hemodialysis?" And, because they did not consider and explore her life context as it related to her clinical presentation—recurrent ER visits for missed hemodialysis with life-threatening physiologic changes—they did not explore what they might be able to do to assist her in circumventing those obstacles. Although they got the technical, or biomedical, aspects of her care right each time she came to the hospital, it took numerous admissions before they explored the context, enabling her finally to manage multiple competing critical life priorities.

Blinders to context are evident in the term Ms. Garcia's doctors used to account for her missing her dialysis: she was "noncompliant." When patients do not stick to a care plan, doctors often conclude they are "noncompliant." The inference is that they are willfully not following instructions. This label is likely to lead to sermonizing about how they need to do better. Consider an alternative term, one that we prefer: "nonadherent." To say someone is nonadherent is merely to describe a behavior that calls for an explanation. What are the possible reasons they are not adhering to the care plan? To answer that question requires exploring context.

What constitutes "context" when caring for patients? A patient's context may be defined as everything expressed outside the skin that is relevant to planning their care. It is an all-encompassing concept that includes not only practical considerations—such as whether a patient has transportation or competing responsibilities, as in the case of Ms. Garcia—but all the cultural and social dimensions of an individual's life that may have an impact on how they view themselves as a patient and how they regard those who provide them care.

Here is another example: Jake Sayer went to his pediatrician for a high school sports physical. Dr. Barry Cohn was a tall man, probably in his late fifties, with short, thick salt and pepper hair. As Dr. Cohn was leaving the exam room at the end of the visit, he peered down at Jake over his spectacles and proclaimed sadly, "Young man, I'm afraid you're not going to grow any taller." That was the first time Jake had heard his 5'5 ½" height portrayed as a misfortune. It had never struck him as a problem. However, that comment and look from his doctor told him that from the vantage point of an expert, things had not quite worked out well. Jake said that after that encounter, he began to think of his height as a problem.

The incident started with an assumption by Dr. Cohn that, for a male, being short is a problem, and that he just owed it to the young man to deliver a hard truth. If, instead, he had realized that short boys can be self-conscious about their stature because of social conventions, and that this can cause distress, he might have asked Jake how he felt about his height. Had he done so, he would have learned that Jake had not been exposed to conventional views about male physique, having grown up without a television, missed a lot of social messaging, and been raised in a family that prized scholarly achievement rather than physical stature.

In both these examples, the clinicians' failures to explore context were coupled with assumptions they made to fill in the gaps in their knowledge—assumptions that reflected their personal perspectives. For Ms. Garcia it was, essentially, that sometimes people just do not take good care of themselves and need to be reminded to get it together. For Jake, it was that being short is a misfortune and that good doctors should be truthful but show some sympathy. In both instances, an assumption was substituted for asking a question.

Placing patients in buckets that fit the doctor's view of the world plays out in physician–patient encounters in myriad ways: Our friend Rebecca recently decided to leave her cardiologist because of an assumption that the doctor made about her eating habits. Rebecca is overweight despite the fact that she follows a Mediterranean diet and exercises daily. Her doctor, after noting that her cholesterol was fine, said she just needed to lose weight and handed her a packet of information on healthy eating to take home with her. The instructions were not news to Rebecca: avoid fast food restaurants, sugary soda drinks, high-fat recipes, etc. Rather than questioning Rebecca about her diet and eating habits, the doctor had assumed a set of behaviors that did not apply in this situation. Rebecca felt like she had been stereotyped and, indeed, it seems like she had been. What the doctor had failed to do was to consider how Rebecca's particular life situation—her context—might be essential to managing her obesity. As Rebecca put it, "My problem is that I eat too much of all the right foods, and I don't know how to control how much I eat." Rebecca concluded that she was receiving poor advice because her doctor had not made an effort to get to know her.

STUDYING PHYSICIAN DECISION-MAKING: THE IMPORTANCE OF EXAMINING THE MUNDANE

Discussions of how doctors think and how they communicate fall primarily into two broad categories: First, much has been said about how doctors miss important diagnoses because of their cognitive biases or lack of powers of observation. The argument is that great doctors are great diagnosticians because they are more methodical, more patient, ask more open-ended questions, listen better, and set aside their assumptions, all to uncover the rare disease. These are the behaviors of exceptional diagnosticians puzzling out rare conditions. Our interest, however, is in a problem that is more mundane but more pervasive, resulting in daily failures to provide patients with competent care. Missing rare diagnoses is rare, because rare conditions, by definition, do not appear very often, and medical technology has made the inner workings and malfunctions of the body ever more transparent. The challenge in the bread-and-butter day-to-day practice of medicine is not answering questions like, "Does this patient have porphyria cutanea tarda?" but "What can I do to help this patient get her diabetes and high blood pressure under control?" When a patient says, for instance, "Boy, it's been tough since I lost my job," does the doctor recognize this as a clue as to why the patient has lost control of his blood pressure? Does the doctor ask, "How has it been difficult since you lost your job?" and discover that the patient can no longer afford the brand-name antihypertensive cardio-selective beta blocker he was prescribed? Does the doctor use this information to prescribe a cheaper generic?

The second broad category concerns physicians' poor interactive communication skills: that they are often insensitive, do not listen well, interrupt, and impose their plan of care. Again, we do not dispute the prevalence of poor communication behavior, which has been documented in numerous studies. What we believe is needed, however, is an understanding of how specific communication behaviors measurably improve or undermine care. Consider, for instance, a clinician's possible responses to that comment by their patient, "Boy, it's been tough since I lost my job." A widely used tool for evaluating physician communication behavior, the Roter Interaction Analysis System, or RIAS[1], categorizes the response, "Yes, the job market has been really awful lately. I'm sorry you are having such a hard time," favorably, as empathic and patient centered. Although it is gratifying that the doctor validates the patient's feelings of struggle, the response also represents a missed opportunity to uncover how lapsed insurance coverage for a drug the patient is taking is the cause of the patient's loss of control over his chronic condition. In sum, the research on communication has produced measures of communication behavior, but has not shed light on how that behavior specifically affects whether patients receive the health care they need.

In our work as educators of medical students and residents, we have seen repeatedly how physicians' views of their roles and responsibilities, when limited to a narrow technical focus that is blind to context, can undermine care. As researchers studying the problem, we have described the phenomenon as "inattention to patient context," because the behavior reflects a failure to consider what might or might not be going on in the life and in the mind of the person for whom we are caring.

Our aim in this book is to share what we have learned about how physicians succeed or fail at taking patient context into account when planning care. In addition, we describe *how* we have learned about attention to context in our research. Initially, we collected many anecdotes based on observations or reports of encounters between patients and residents. Residents are physicians in their own right who are still in a supervised phase of their training. As a result, they are observed and scrutinized in a manner that independently practicing physicians are not. As such, the care they provide is easier to document.

Once we began conducting formal research, we found that attending physicians are prone to the same habits of mind as residents. Systematically studying physician cognitive behavior required unconventional methods, such as employing professional actors to work as undercover patients and recruiting real patients to record their encounters covertly.

FAULTING THE PATIENT: THE FUNDAMENTAL ATTRIBUTION ERROR

Inattention to context represents a lack of curiosity. It may be due, in part, to what psychologists refer to as the "fundamental attribution error," which is, essentially, a failure to consider the complex situational reasons other people may behave irrationally or inappropriately, and instead attributing their behavior to a fundamental flaw in their character.[2] This is likely the reason why the healthcare team responsible for Ms. Garcia did not think to ask, "Why in the world is this woman, who seems reasonably intelligent, coming to an unpleasant place—our ER—so often for a problem that is easy to avoid?" Interestingly, the fundamental attribution error is not one that we make when thinking about ourselves, because we are in an excellent position to see the relevance of context to our own lives. Ms. Garcia had no difficulty explaining why she was missing her hemodialysis. She only needed to be asked. Perhaps because she was unaware that there were things the healthcare team could do to help her, and perhaps because of the language barrier, she never volunteered the information.

When the fundamental attribution error leads doctors to focus on patient personality rather than life context, it can lead to misunderstandings that may have serious consequences for the patient. A resident physician described his patient, Melanie Davis, as "anti-social" to his supervising attending, noting that she did not even acknowledge him when he came into the exam room. When the attending subsequently entered, he extended his hand in greeting to Ms. Davis who was perched on an exam table and, sure enough, she did not reciprocate. Initially, the attending did not say anything and proceeded with the interaction, noticing along the way that she seemed pleasant. Near the end of the visit, he asked her why she had not taken his hand when he had entered and offered it to her. Initially, she looked puzzled. It turned out, however, that she had lost her peripheral vision several years earlier from a pituitary tumor that had been removed, and the door through which the doctor entered and approached her was outside her field of vision. The resident's assessment that the patient was unfriendly reflected an ingrained association between a social convention (the handshake) and an individual's personal qualities. The resident did not question the discrepancy between the patient's apparently rude behavior and her otherwise genial demeanor. Had the discrepancy not been explored with a simple question, her doctors would have regarded her as disengaged, a perception that could have shaped how they related to her, potentially undermining her care.

The tendency toward judging a patient's behavior instead of exploring its context leads to many false conclusions—including that a patient is not responsible (Garcia), that she is rude (Davis), or in the following example that he is "demanding." What physicians experience as demands, patients may intend as an expression of need. This perception persists because it accounts for a lot of patient behavior from the perspective of the doctor making the assumption. That does not mean, however, that the assumption is valid. Patients come to doctors with needs. They may express those needs indirectly as specific requests. A patient who is suffering from chronic back pain may say "Doctor, I've got to have some Vicodin for my pain," because he has heard that this particular (often abused) medication works for pain. The doctor interprets the request as "demanding" or "drug seeking" when it is really just a call for help—and that call goes unanswered as the physician lectures the patient on why narcotics are not appropriate for treating chronic pain but neglects to explore the patient's job responsibilities with heavy lifting.

Sometimes it seems as if physicians go to great lengths to avoid asking questions about context. The rationalization that patients are "just demanding," for instance, can extend to situations where the drug sought is not even pleasant. Consider Mr. Eli Gates, an African-American Vietnam veteran in his sixties, who came in with his wife requesting antibiotics for what he believed was an infected tooth. He was seen initially by Dr. Jennifer Carter, a resident physician who had seen him a couple of times before. After meeting and examining the patient, Dr. Carter came out of the exam room to explain to her attending, Dr. Suresh Mehta, that she did not see any signs of an abscess, but Mr. Gates's teeth were generally in terrible shape and he badly needed to see a dentist. She said that she explained this to her patient, but he insisted that he just needed antibiotics. She said that he was demanding them despite her best efforts, and that they were at an impasse over the issue.

When Dr. Mehta entered the exam room, he saw a man in a wheelchair, but noted that he did not appear to be frail or ill. Dr. Mehta extended his hand and got the bone crushing handshake typical of sturdy older veterans. Peering into Mr. Gates's mouth, he confirmed Dr. Carter's findings: lots of severe tooth decay and inflamed gums but nothing red-hot, no signs of an abscess. Despite his repetition of Dr. Carter's assessment to Mr. Gates, the patient insisted that he did not need to see a dentist. At one point, when Drs. Carter and Mehta were looking up options for scheduling him in the dental clinic on the computer, Mr. Gates turned to his wife and said, "Let's just get out of here. They're no help." His wife did not budge. She said nothing.

Feeling his only option was to educate Mr. Gates, Dr. Mehta was about to give him a lecture on how antibiotics are not the answer to everything. His curiosity kicked in, however, and instead he asked a question, partially prompted by noticing that the patient's wife did not seem to be on the same page as her husband: "Why are you saying we are no help, when you can see that we are trying to help you?" There was a long pause during which Mr. Gates did not say anything. He just stared at the floor. Then his wife said, "He's afraid of needles. He won't go to the dentist because of the needles."

Dr. Mehta asked Mr. Gates how long he had been afraid of needles and why. Mr. Gates answered that it had started when he was a kid in the 1950s and got a polio shot. He said the people administering the shots reused the needles, and between injections they sterilized them in a flame. In his case, they had not waited for the needle to cool, so he got an injection with a red-hot and probably dull needle. He was sufficiently traumatized by that experience that he had avoided needles at all costs throughout adulthood, including visits to the dentist. Dr. Mehta wondered how many other poor kids from that era were similarly mistreated.

The conversation quickly transitioned to a frank discussion about traumatic experience and desensitization therapy as a treatment for his phobia. Mr. Gates acknowledged that he had not talked about it before, and that no one had asked. The poor state of his mouth was a testament to a lifetime of fearing and avoiding preventive dental care. Perhaps most importantly, the tone of the interaction changed dramatically. Mr. Gates dropped his request for antibiotics, and his bitterness about not being helped dissipated.

ANOTHER REASON TO CONTEXTUALIZE CARE: LOWER COSTS

Not only can inattention to context be deleterious to patient health, it also may drive up costs by leading to unnecessary care. Ms. Garcia's multiple emergency room visits are certainly an example of that. Two other patients one of us wrote about in papers published in 2004 experienced "near misses" in which costly and inappropriate care was narrowly averted with attention to context.[3,4] The first case concerned Bette Wilson, who at age 59 was living with hypertension, diabetes, overweight, and recent shortness of breath and fatigue. The resident, Dr. Patrick Gideon, who took the medical history and conducted the initial exam, related to the supervising attending that the symptoms had worsened over the last eight months and were relieved with rest. He also mentioned that she had smoked a pack of cigarettes a day for 10 years when she was in her twenties and thirties. In light of all these risk factors, Dr. Gideon thought he needed to determine if she had heart disease, emphysema, asthma, congestive heart failure, hypothyroidism, or chronic pulmonary emboli. He ticked off a list of imaging studies and blood tests he planned to order. As the attending headed toward the exam room to meet the patient, it was hard to disagree with the proposed plan, which seemed prudent, albeit extensive, given that it would require cardiac ultrasound, CT scanning, and nuclear imaging.

Entering the exam room, the attending physician encountered a petite but overweight woman with a soft handshake and polite smile. Ms. Wilson recalled longstanding efforts to improve her health, including her success at quitting smoking 25 years ago, followed by less success controlling her weight until quite recently. She described embarking on an exercise program with a friend a couple of years ago, and how she had begun to feel much better after losing considerable weight and becoming quite fit. She had come to enjoy shopping on foot rather than driving everywhere, was generally in a better mood, and had stopped feeling short of breath or fatigued when she exerted herself. Unfortunately, however, the gains she had made were recently lost when her friend and exercise buddy left town to care for a grandchild in another state following a daughter's recent divorce. Ms. Wilson acknowledged that she had returned to her sedentary ways, and with that regression, her excess weight had returned as had her prior signs and symptoms of being out of shape.

With a few questions, the attending confirmed that the disappearance followed by reappearance of her symptoms coincided with initiation and disengagement from the long walks and activities at a fitness center that Ms. Wilson had participated in for about a year. The discovery that Ms. Wilson's medical complaints had resolved with a bit of exercise and companionship and then returned when she relapsed into a sedentary lifestyle ruled out the physiologic causes that Dr. Gideon planned to run tests to evaluate. Much expense, inconvenience, and a possible cascade of testing leading to more and increasingly invasive testing could be avoided. The discovery also pointed to a new treatment strategy: helping Ms. Wilson get back into another exercise program. The biggest challenge, Ms. Wilson acknowledged, seemed to be finding another person she liked who would motivate her to become active again. They discussed several options for finding exercise buddies, and agreed that Ms. Wilson would return in a few weeks to provide an update on her plan.

The second case involved Thelma Dawson, who at the time was 44 years old, weighed 270 pounds, and was struggling to lose weight. She was planning to have bariatric surgery, a weight-reduction surgery in which portions of the stomach and small intestine are bypassed. Dr. Chou, the attending internist staffing the preoperative testing clinic, met her while supervising a small team of residents who saw all patients initially. Ms. Dawson's record indicated that her primary care doctor had referred her to a multidisciplinary obesity weight-loss center where she had participated in a diet and exercise program before seeing a bariatric surgeon. Indications for bariatric surgery at the time included a body mass index greater than 34, previous unsuccessful attempts at weight loss, and medical complications attributable to obesity. Ms. Dawson's complications were diabetes and high blood pressure.

The resident, Dr. Benjamin, who saw Ms. Dawson, ticked off all of her indications for surgery to Dr. Chou, reporting that her physical exam was unremarkable and that a screening electrocardiogram was normal. One complicating factor, however, was documented in a note by the surgeon who had referred her to the preoperative testing clinic. Ms. Dawson previously had had gallbladder surgery, which meant that she likely had scar tissue—"adhesions"—in her abdomen. As a result the surgery could not be conducted laparoscopically through a tiny hole. Instead, the procedure would require a conventional approach, meaning that Ms. Dawson would have to recover from a large incision, which would take much longer. Dr. Benjamin mentioned that he had discussed all this with Ms. Dawson, but she had replied that she still wanted the procedure. Offhandedly, he mentioned her comment that one reason she was eager to lose weight was to be able to take better care of a chronically ill son. Curious, Dr. Chou asked what was wrong with Ms. Dawson's son. Dr. Benjamin replied that he had no idea but had concluded that as far as the patient was concerned, she was low-risk and an operative intervention seemed appropriate. It all sounded pretty straightforward: the reasons for weight reduction surgery were clear, the patient was informed, and she had personal motivating factors to have it done.

When Dr. Chou met Ms. Dawson a few minutes later in the exam room, she asked the patient about her son. Ms. Dawson explained that James was 22 years old and had progressed to an advanced stage of muscular dystrophy, now requiring assistance with all activities of daily living including toileting and bathing. She physically lifted him from his bed to his wheelchair and from his wheelchair to his bath each morning. It turned out that Ms. Dawson did not have much help and that even when she did, James was only really comfortable with her. Ms. Dawson explained that her husband had a drinking problem and was not reliable. She also had an eight-year-old daughter who depended on her. They went shopping together, and her daughter could be helpful at times, but Ms. Dawson still carried the heavier groceries up two flights of stairs to their apartment on Chicago's north side. Her knees sometimes ached and she anticipated she would manage better with less weight.

One of the challenges of healing from an abdominal wound is avoiding any heavy lifting for several weeks. For patients recovering from open (i.e., not laparoscopic) bariatric surgery, the rule is to avoid straining abdominal muscles for five to six weeks. Failure to adhere—particularly during the first week or so—can result in reopening the wound, which causes pain, an increased risk of infection, a need for more surgery, and prolonged healing.

Drs. Benjamin and Chou explained to Ms. Dawson that she would not be able to safely lift or bathe her son or carry heavy groceries for at least a month following surgery. As they discussed her home situation, Ms. Dawson expressed dismay at the implications for her children: "They need me now more than ever," she said. She commented that though she had been informed by the surgeon about the postoperative course, she had been so focused on the positive aspects of surgery, particularly greater mobility, that she had not really thought it through. She concluded, and they concurred, that this was the wrong time for the procedure. She cancelled surgery.

How serious are such mistakes if they are not prevented by a member of the care team who is attentive to context? Sending Ms. Dawson to the operating room for an elective surgical procedure when she could not have complied with instructions for a safe postoperative recovery would have set her up for complications that were otherwise preventable. Had this occurred, and had she returned to the hospital with an open wound requiring additional surgery and further risk of complications such as infection, would it have occurred to anyone that the problem could have been prevented had there been greater consideration in advance of her life situation, or context? Or would the physicians simply have reported that Ms. Dawson was "noncompliant" with instructions not to do any heavy lifting when she returned home?

CONTEXTUALIZING CARE: WHAT DOES IT TAKE?

Healthcare providers like lists because they are useful tools for remembering what to think about in a particular situation. At the heart of medical training is the "differential diagnosis," or "differential," as it is often abbreviated. The differential is a list of all the various biomedical conditions that could account for a particular cluster of signs and symptoms. For instance, the differential for chest pain and shortness of breath would include heart attack, pneumonia, and an anxiety disorder, along with several more obscure conditions.

The challenge of attending to context is that everyone's life is complicated and different. What kinds of things are essential to know about another person in order to provide appropriate care? Specifically, what is the "relevant context"? For Ms. Garcia, the relevant context was her ill son and the problems she was having with transportation to her appointments. If one were to create categories, one could think of these as, respectively, "competing responsibilities" and "access to care." Mrs. Dawson's relevant context would also fall under the category of competing responsibilities and, additionally, a lack of "social support." For Mr. Gates, providing contextually appropriate care required knowing about his relationship with his healthcare providers, and the origins of his distrust dating back to a traumatic experience with needles. Based on these and many other cases, we identified 10 broad domains of patient context: *access to care, social support, competing responsibilities, financial situation, relationship with healthcare providers, skills and abilities, emotional state, cultural/spiritual beliefs, environment,* and *attitude toward illness.* Our 10 domains of patient context can be thought of as a "contextual differential" for patients presenting with symptoms (what the patient feels) or signs (what the doctor observes) that may be attributable to their life circumstances.

It is likely that nearly all of us have circumstances in our lives that have implications for our health care; some of the time we are personally aware of what those contextual issues are. For instance, if we have lost the ability to pay for medication that is not covered by our health plan, we know that to be a problem. We may be ashamed, however, to mention it to our doctor. In other instances, we are not prepared to acknowledge a problem to ourselves, even when it is obvious to others who are close to us. Although Mr. Gates was not ready to volunteer the information about his underlying trauma and phobia with needles, his wife knew why he was insisting on antibiotics when what he really needed was a dentist. Finally, there are times when we have nothing to hide but simply do not have the medical knowledge to make the connection between our life situation and our health care. That was the case for Ms. Dawson, who knew what she needed to do for her dependent children, but did not appreciate how the surgery would keep her from meeting those obligations.

Because patients find it difficult to connect the dots between their healthcare needs and their life context on their own, they need a close collaboration with their physician. Although there is much that an astute patient can do to alert a clinician to the relevance of context to care, it is fundamentally the physician's job to understand the need for such collaboration and to consistently take the initiative to ensure it happens. Imagine an elderly relative or friend who begins to decline because of changes caused by early Alzheimer's disease. If he has been living independently, the deterioration may undermine his ability to take his medications. If he has diabetes, his blood sugars may become critically elevated, or if he is confused enough to take too much medication, dangerously low. It is unrealistic to expect him to recognize that his confusion is causing his diabetes to get out of control. That is the doctor's job.

When doctors are not thinking broadly about context when considering why a disease may be getting worse, they are by default thinking narrowly about the disease process as a biomedical problem. Their focus is on the physiology exclusive of the surrounding context. For instance, type 2 diabetes—the most common type—often naturally progresses as patients get older because of changes that occur in the responsiveness of bodily tissues to insulin. The management for progressive diabetes often involves overcoming progressive insulin "insensitivity" with higher dosages. Although it is true that diabetes progresses in most patients, it is also true that there are other reasons for progression besides age, and that considering them requires looking beyond the disease to the broader context. A clinician who thinks contextually is not doing so at the expense of thinking about the physiology, but in addition to it. That breadth of thinking is reflected in a broader differential that includes the contextual domains. The clinician who considers the domain of "skills and abilities," for instance, will look for and find deficits on cognitive testing suggesting that a new diagnosis—dementia—has emerged and must be addressed both as a biomedical problem and as a key part of the context of the patient's worsening control of their diabetes.

What does it take to think contextually? Is medical education simply failing to teach students to consider a broader differential when they evaluate disease, one that includes domains of context? That is likely a part of it, but the following anecdote related by a colleague, Dr. Auster, about his experience observing a second-year medical student learning to interview a patient, suggests there is a more fundamental problem:

The patient was a 62-year-old man, hospitalized for the past week, who had been recruited the previous day to meet for a practice interview. At the time he seemed in good spirits and expressed eagerness to assist. However, when we arrived that morning, he seemed distracted. As the student began to question him he responded tersely and with little interest. The student nevertheless forged ahead, trying to make his way through each component of a medical history. As the student struggled, the atmosphere in the room became increasingly oppressive. I finally considered it imperative to intervene: 'Mr. Jones, you seem very upset. Is there something bothering you?' The patient explained that he was told the evening before that he would be discharged that afternoon, and he had arranged for a friend to take him home, but shortly before we arrived, he learned he would have to stay at least another day. He felt some urgency about notifying his friend who would have to leave work early to get to the hospital on time, and he had not yet been able to leave a message or reach him despite trying several numbers. However, he did not want to break his commitment to meet with the student. I said that reaching his friend was the more urgent need, and that other arrangements could be made for the student. The patient's tense demeanor at once dissolved. He shook our hands as we left, and reached for his phone.

As soon as we left the room the student looked at me in amazement and exclaimed 'Wow. How did you do that? I tried so hard to connect with him and you knew what to say immediately.' I replied 'If he had been your friend looking that upset, wouldn't you have asked him the same question?' As if a light bulb had suddenly gone on, the student exclaimed 'You mean you talk to patients like you talk to people?'

The student's genuine surprise reveals a problem that extends well beyond this student and this particular story. Something is missing, not only in the lists of things budding physicians are taught to ask about, but in their conception of their relationship to the person they come to think of as a "patient." The patient is perceived as someone upon whom a set of tasks must be completed, rather than as a person with whom one seeks to engage. Simply broadening that list of tasks to include interrogating patients about their life situation, without engaging with the patient to uncover the underlying problem, is not enough.

CONTEXTUALIZING CARE: FROM CHECKLISTS TO ENGAGEMENT

The importance of engagement is evident when making nuanced assessments of patients that go beyond following guidelines or completing checklists. Consider, for instance, the evaluation of patients who may want to kill themselves. One well-trained resident, Dr. Sheila Bentham, knew to ask a series of questions about suicidal thoughts and plans when her patient, Mr. Beasly, commented that he had stopped taking all his medication because he "might just end it all." She asked him if he had other plans for ending his life, including whether he kept a gun in the home; he said he did not. Nevertheless, Dr. Bentham was understandably concerned and shared with her attending supervisor, Dr. Creager, that perhaps they should refer the patient to psychiatry for an immediate and more comprehensive evaluation. Dr. Bentham had completed a set of tasks yielding some useful information, but did not know how to engage with Mr. Beasly.

As Dr. Creager entered the exam room he offered Mr. Beasly a fist bump instead of a handshake, explaining that he was a guitarist and trying to protect his slightly arthritic hands. Mr. Beasly smiled, saying, "That's cool. I understand." Dr. Creager seated himself on the exam table so he could face Mr. Beasly, who was in a chair near the desk where the resident sat at a computer. Dr. Creager began, "Mr. Beasly, I understand you have been feeling down and are not taking your medications. Is that correct? Tell me what's going on." In the dialogue that followed, Dr. Creager learned about Mr. Beasly's decades of struggle with post-traumatic stress disorder (PTSD) dating back to his service in Vietnam in the late 1960s and early 1970s. He learned that Mr. Beasly also had a successful 30-year marriage with a wife who cared for him deeply and whom he trusted completely to keep an eye on him and help him stay sane. He noted Mr. Beasly's high degree of self-knowledge, how he had learned to avoid PTSD triggers such as being on buses, in tunnels ("reminds me of chasing after Viet Cong in their sandals in black dark tunnels in Saigon," he said with a shudder), or in crowded public places alone, where flashbacks and intense paranoia were easily triggered. At one point during the conversation, when Mr. Beasly was relating his struggles with claustrophobia, he pointed toward the shut door and said, "Being in small rooms like this with the doors closed can freak me out." Dr. Creager interjected. "Would you like me to open the door a crack for you?"

Mr. Beasly replied, "No, that's not necessary. I am feeling cared for now as you all have your attention on my health, so I'm not feeling at all like I need to get out of here. I'm feeling pretty good." During the encounter, which lasted about seven minutes, Dr. Creager began to feel connected to Mr. Beasly and felt a sense of pleasure and relief at the resilience of the man he was beginning to know. After asking a few more questions to see if Mr. Beasly had any tendencies towards impulsive self-destructive behavior—and determining he did not—he felt comfortable with a plan that Mr. Beasly would follow up with Dr. Bentham and Dr. Creager, as well as with psychiatry in a few weeks, and would call sooner if he had any concerns. Mr. Beasly, who had not seen a physician in some time, seemed appreciative and relaxed at the end of the visit, and Dr. Creager felt confident that he was going to do OK.

After Mr. Beasly had left, Dr. Creager asked Dr. Bentham what she had learned during the encounter. Dr. Bentham, who struck Dr. Creager as a particularly bright and conscientious young physician, thought for a moment and said, "There were some questions you asked that I had not thought of and should have known to consider. Also, I liked the way you offered to open the door when he said he had claustrophobia." Pushing a bit further, Dr. Creager said, "That's good . . . but I'm wondering did you get any sense of the man during my discussions with him that you found helpful?" Dr. Bentham stared blankly, looking somewhat puzzled, unsure what to say. Dr. Creager followed gently with "Sheila, do you have an idea of what it is I am asking?" "No, I don't think so," she replied. Dr. Creager went on to share his impressions of Mr. Beasly as someone who had strong social support, who knew himself well, and who was capable of connecting with other people. Because of these qualities, Dr. Creager related, he did not seem in danger of committing a violent act either to himself or to others. Although each of these observations was the product of a question Dr. Creager had asked, there had been no checklist. It had started with a fist bump followed by two people sitting together trying to solve a problem. The encounter had felt satisfying to Dr. Creager, and nourishing. For Mr. Beasly it felt healing. And a contextually appropriate care plan had emerged from the interaction.

RESEARCH ON CONTEXTUALIZATION OF CARE: FROM ANECDOTE TO SYSTEMATIC STUDY

These are true stories (although we have changed the names of the patients and physicians). We find these accounts compelling. But we are researchers, and stories are not proof of a generalized phenomenon, nor do they document the scope or magnitude of what is observed. The idea that attention to context is essential to care planning for many patients may be regarded as a hypothesis. It is a possible explanation for why so many patients do not benefit from treatments that have been demonstrated in studies to be effective. Although each example of the adverse impact of inattention to context builds a case for the importance of contextualizing care, one cannot draw general conclusions from anecdotes.

In considering how to test our hypothesis we realized we would have to ask and answer several questions: How could we measure attention to relevant patient context? To do so we would need a precise definition of "relevant patient context" and a strategy for deciding whether the clinician had attended to it (and how that would be defined). Whatever definitions we settled upon would require measurement tools and strategies, and those tools and strategies would need to be both accurate and reliable, meaning that they were measuring what they were supposed to be measuring, and that they could be counted on to deliver the same results regardless of when or by whom the measures were employed.

With tools like these, we could begin to explore several questions: First, when relevant patient context—meaning information specific to a particular patient's life situation that is relevant to planning appropriate care—is present in an encounter, how often do physicians notice and address the context in their care plan? Second, in what proportion of encounters does care hinge on identifying and addressing relevant patient context? Third—and perhaps most importantly—what are the implications for the patient's healthcare outcomes if the contextually relevant information is, or is not, addressed in their care plan?

In addition to these foundational questions about frequency and impact, three other questions also seemed important to explore: First, health care in most countries is a substantial expense for both the patient and society, and policymakers are increasingly concerned not only with quality of care but the cost and value of that care. What are the cost implications of attending or not attending to context? Second, in which of the 10 domains of context are physicians more or less likely to find and address contextual factors in care planning? And, finally, is attention to context teachable? Specifically, can physicians learn to notice when things do not add up and respond with curiosity and engagement rather than assumptions or inattention? In the following chapters, we answer these questions.

Measuring the Problem

"Doctor, things have been tough since I lost my job."
"I'm sorry to hear that. Do you have any allergies?"
—*Transcript of hidden audio-recording between*
an undercover actor and a doctor

A s noted in Chapter 1, doctors are pretty good at attending to the routine biomedical aspects of care, but run into difficulty when the individual differences in patients' lives—their context—calls for variation from the routine. Doctors follow guidelines even when there are clues that those guidelines may not apply. A major part of the problem seems to be inattention to context due in part to the Fundamental Attribution Error, common both in and outside the profession of medicine. The training and culture of medical practice, however, adds additional obstacles, and one of them is an emphasis on standardizing everything, a perspective that is anathema to a consideration of context. To understand the push for standardizing care, and why doctors would do this, it is helpful to look back a few decades.

VARIATIONS IN CARE: WHAT YOU GET DEPENDS
ON WHOM YOU SEE

In the 1960s and 1970s, researchers became concerned about a problem in
health care: Different physicians often recommended different treatments
for the same diseases and conditions. That could make sense because different physicians treated different patients—an endocrinologist seeing
a relatively healthy patient in an urban area might treat diabetes differently than a general internist treating a patient with other health issues
in a rural area. Some treatments affect men and women or members of
different racial groups differently, and it is important to consider such
factors in order to treat patients appropriately. (Although studies have
also demonstrated that sometimes, due to conscious or unconscious bias,
physicians have prescribed different treatments to patients of different
sexes or races even when the same treatment would be recommended.)
Researchers call differences in the kinds of patients seen by a physician
"case mix." But study after study found that even after controlling for
case mix and other factors like sex and race, physicians made different
treatment decisions for similar disorders. In many cases, it seemed like
one treatment was better than another, and so some physicians must have
been practicing incorrectly even as they thought they were doing the right
thing. If evidence strongly suggests that a particular treatment is best for
a condition—for example, that heart attack patients should receive prescriptions for beta blocker drugs to prevent further attacks—and some
physicians are not providing that treatment, their patients are receiving
inadequate care and may be suffering unnecessarily.

In the 1980s, two movements in medicine emerged in response to
this concern about variation. The first, evidence-based medicine (EBM),
urged physicians to learn how to find and evaluate the quality of research
evidence (usually published in papers in medical journals). This enabled
doctors to determine which treatments were proven to be most effective
and then provide those treatments to their patients. By offering tools and
training, EBM advocates hoped that different physicians would agree
on the same evidence, draw the same conclusions, and select the same

treatments. EBM remains an important component of medical education in the United States and other countries, and we will return to it in our discussion of medical education in Chapter 6.

The second movement was the development of clinical practice guidelines (CPGs). A clinical practice guideline is a recommendation, issued by a group of physicians or medical researchers, acting on behalf of an organization or national institution, for how physicians should treat or diagnose groups of patients with a particular condition. For example, guidelines suggest which tests should be administered, and in what order, to diagnose a condition that is hard to observe (such as Down syndrome in a fetus), particularly when some of the tests are potentially harmful. The influential U.S. Institute of Medicine issued a report recommending clinical practice guidelines in 1990, and a follow-up report with further suggestions on how to improve the development and adoption of guidelines in 2011.[1,2]

Most clinical practice guidelines are issued by medical societies or government agencies, such as the National Institute for Health and Care Excellence (NICE) in the United Kingdom or the Preventive Services Task Force in the United States. Guideline developers typically define a group of patients, review evidence for treatment options, make a series of recommendations, and indicate the strength of the recommendations and the quality of the evidence backing them. Clinical practice guidelines seemed like a simple solution to the problem of performance variation—let experts review the evidence and tell physicians what they recommend. If the guidelines are clear, and physicians adopt and implement the guidelines, their decisions about similar patients should be the same, right? And if those guidelines really reflect the best evidence, making the same decisions for similar patients should lead to better health. Today, clinical practice guidelines are ubiquitous.

Of course, just because patients may be similar, it does not mean they are identical. Although guidelines explain how best to help a group of patients overall, some individual patients in the group may not be receiving appropriate care under clinical practice guidelines. A medical error is a specific instance of inappropriate care. The study of medical error has been a major focus of 21st century health care. An Institute of Medicine (IOM) report issued in 2000, *To Err is Human: Building a Safer Health System,*[3] brought the issue to the forefront and drew the attention of medical professionals and policymakers. The report found that as many as 100,000 Americans die each year due to medical errors—more than due to car accidents, breast cancer, or AIDS—and that these errors are largely preventable through improved systems of prescribing and double-checking.

The IOM report adopted a definition of error based on the work of the psychologist James Reason in his book *Human Error.*[4] Error is "the failure of a planned action to be completed as intended (i.e., error of execution) or the use of a wrong plan to achieve an aim (i.e., error of planning)." The IOM report reviewed dozens of studies of medical error. Nearly all of the studies document either errors during hospitalization (such as surgical injuries, patient misidentification, and hospital-related infections) or medication errors (wrong dosages, prescribing medications the patient is known to be allergic to, and contraindicated combinations of drugs). A sizable fraction of these errors are diagnostic errors, in which physicians delayed testing, chose the wrong test, or ignored test results. Medical errors often can be detected through review of patient medical records once the patient's correct diagnosis and treatment are known, or once the patient has been discharged from the hospital (a patient is unlikely to be discharged from the hospital without a definite diagnosis and plan, and the chart ought to record all the medications and procedures the patient received), or, regrettably, through death certificates and autopsy records.

CONTEXTUAL ERROR: THE HIDDEN SIDE OF MEDICAL ERROR

For decades, faculty at academic medical centers have been teaching their residents EBM and making sure they have access to the most up-to-date guidelines. Likewise, hospitals increasingly have instituted patient safety programs focused on reducing medical error. Anyone who has been in a hospital recently has probably noticed some of these programs. For example, patients may be surprised at how often they are asked to provide a name and another piece of identifying information (like a birthdate) to ensure that they are not receiving drugs or treatments meant for a patient in another room. They also may have noticed signs inviting patients to ask their doctors to wash their hands, an important guideline to reduce the spread of hospital-acquired infection.

The University of Illinois Medical Center taught EBM, encouraged the use of guidelines, and implemented patient safety programs. Residents were highly skilled at identifying medical problems and well-versed in the clinical practice guidelines for common internal medicine conditions and treatments. They regularly applied guidelines and prescribed evidence-based treatments for their patients.

And yet, we began to see a problematic pattern among our residents and their patients. The problem was that these guidelines did not make sense for patients whose contextual factors were not typical. When residents did not discover these contextual factors, they did not know that the treatment guidelines needed to be modified. Consequently, they made a contextual error—they prescribed the "right treatment" for the wrong patient. They missed the patient's true diagnosis (an error of planning) or failed to realize that contextual factors prevented the patient from carrying out the recommended treatment (an error of execution).

We had read papers about how physicians overlooked psychosocial issues in patient care. But none of these studies were designed to provide scientific evidence that doctors could harm patients by not paying attention to their life situation, nor were they designed to discover how often physicians might make these mistakes.

So how does one identify contextual errors? This is a surprisingly difficult problem, because the medical record alone is of no help. Consider a doctor seeing a patient for unexplained weight loss who mentions that he no longer has family in the area. Concerned about cancer, the doctor, following standards of care, orders a battery of tests to assess the likelihood and extent of malignancy. Another physician, more knowledgeable about mental health, reviews the patient's history, symptoms, normal physical exam, and concludes that the patient was instead depressed and had stopped eating. The initial diagnosis was wrong, and had the patient committed suicide before the cancer workup returned negative, it would have been a preventable death from a medical error. In this case, a review of the chart could identify the error.

But what if both physicians were wrong? How would we know? What if the underlying issue was not cancer or depression (both biomedical factors), but lack of food, a contextual factor that affects as many as one in seven households in the United States?* In this instance, the medical record would show symptoms that suggest cancer, justifying the physician's plan. But because the patient did not have access to food, the plan is wrong. If the patient had suffered complications from a biopsy, this would have been a preventable bad outcome. A review of the chart would not identify that an error had been made.

Hospitals, insurance companies, researchers, and regulatory agencies commonly use medical record review to assess physician performance and to identify error. The fundamental problem is that medical records do not show what the physician does not know—or knows but does not consider. If the physician did not notice or explore the patient's comment about no longer having family in the area, the only clue that he is alone and hungry, she would not have recorded it in the chart. If we review that chart, we will see a physician make what looks like correct decisions about workup and treatment based on the medical history and the physical exam she conducted and recorded. From the chart alone, there is no way to see the contextual factor, or identify that a contextual error occurred; we need more insight about the patient than the physician either obtained or considered important enough to enter into the chart.

How about asking the patient? Another important approach to assessing physician performance is patient satisfaction surveys. Hospitals, practice groups, payers, and researchers also regularly employ such surveys

* That statistic comes from the U.S. Department of Agriculture and was reported in a November 17, 2009 *Washington Post* article by Amy Goldstein entitled "Hunger a growing problem in America, USDA reports."

to identify areas of strength and concern. They are an effective way to summarize the experience of groups of patients and to compare the way different doctors' patients experience their health care. We also know, however, that such surveys paint an incomplete picture. They rarely provide enough detail about individual patients to pick out contextual factors. Even if they did, patients may not remember exactly what they told their physician, and are not trained to recognize whether and when their doctor overlooks or fails to record key contextual information in their medical history. Do we expect the malnourished patient to fill out a survey saying that his physician missed his real problem and pursued an unnecessary and potentially hazardous workup? Can he be counted on to recognize and explain those errors?

Patient-completed surveys have other problems. Poorly written questions can mislead or confuse patients, and skew the results of surveys. Perhaps even worse, patients who have had bad experiences are less likely to return, and therefore, their crucial experiences and opinions are less often captured. Those who opt to stay are less inclined to be critical because they become emotionally invested in believing they are getting the best care. Survey researchers call these problems *self-selection biases.* When the patients who respond to a survey about hospital stays are not representative of all the patients who stay in the hospital, their responses may not accurately reflect the experiences of that larger group.

UNANNOUNCED STANDARDIZED PATIENTS: UNCOVERING THE TRUTH

If the chart could not reveal missing patient context, and patients did not know when their context should affect their treatment, we needed a new way to uncover contextual errors. We needed to demonstrate convincingly that even well-trained physicians could miss contextual clues and overlook contextual factors when planning treatment. To provide the strongest proof, we also needed to show that these errors were not about case mix. Our solution was the unannounced standardized patient.

A standardized patient (SP) is a person—often a professional actor—who is trained to consistently portray a patient with a medical problem. Nearly all medical schools now use standardized patients to help train doctors by allowing them to examine important cases that may not arise regularly enough for every student to encounter them. The actors can be trained in what kind of care and communication they should expect, and can provide immediate feedback to the medical student about their performance. Standardized patients are also an important method for assessing the competence of medical students. Many schools include standardized patients as part of their examinations, with scores based on ratings by faculty observers as well as by the standardized patients themselves. The second part of the United States Medical Licensing Examination, which every physician seeking to practice in America must pass to be eligible for licensing, includes a set of 12 standardized patient encounters.

Standardized patients eliminate the problem of case mix in physician performance. The SP plays the same case for each physician they visit. Furthermore, the SP plays the case the same way each time. Every physician seeing the same SP has access to the same facts and opportunity to ask the same questions.

In medical schools, students know when they are examining a standardized patient. Their attention is heightened, and they make efforts to show their best performance. In contrast, unannounced standardized patients (USPs) are standardized patients who present to a real practice, pretending to be a real patient. At the time the doctor examines the USP, the doctor has every reason to believe that the USP is a real patient seeking care—so we have every reason to believe that the doctor's performance will be typical of what she does when she sees real patients (as opposed to a "game day" performance during a known standardized patient encounter).

Other terms that have been used for USPs include "mystery patients" and "secret shoppers." Those terms are easier to say, but are often used when referring to real (unstandardized) patients who report back on things like how easy it is to find the clinic, how long they had to wait to be seen, and other customer service measures, just like secret shoppers visiting retail stores. USPs, in contrast, are standardized and "inside the curtain"—they directly observe the physicians conducting the medical visit.

A few researchers had used unannounced standardized patients for studies, but the numbers of undercover visits were few and the elaborate subterfuge needed to convince doctors across a wide number of practices that they were seeing real patients, not actors in disguise, was daunting. In order to get the USPs into doctors' offices, we would have to create fake medical records, set up fake insurance information, and train actors to both keep to a script and adapt rapidly in response to the doctors, nurses, and medical office staff. We also would have to win the trust and support of the physicians involved, so they would allow themselves to be fooled.

Furthermore, once the USPs were successfully in the doctor's office, how should these undercover visits be structured to collect reliable information about physicians' attention to patient context? USPs collect irrefutable observations when they audio-record the visit, but what would someone look for? These questions brought us together—a primary care physician and a cognitive psychologist trained in the study of medical decision-making and research design—and led us into an extensive dialogue about a variety of strategies for measuring and tracking physician attention to patient contextual information when that attention is critical to proper care. Talking together, we became excited to go beyond the many reports showing that doctors miss psychosocial issues. We set about creating an experimental system to provide the scientific evidence that was missing from previous studies. We would need to isolate and quantify (translate into numbers what had been anecdotal stories) the size of the problem so that it could be systematically analyzed. We came to USPs as a last resort, knowing how difficult it would be to send actors to visit large numbers of doctors, but we realized it was the only way to get the evidence we needed. That decision was the critical turning point in our research.

FAKE PATIENTS + REAL DOCTORS = NEW INSIGHTS

We were not the first to recognize the benefits of using unannounced standardized patients. One of the first published reports using incognito patients was "On being sane in insane places," by D. L. Rosenhan in 1973.[5] In that study, three women and five men visited hospitals pretending to hear voices in their heads in order to get admitted to psychiatric wards. Other than how they described the voices, however, their scripts were not standardized—they talked about events in their own lives. In this respect they were more like the "secret shoppers" who work in retail. Once Rosenhan's "pseudopatients" were admitted, they stopped reporting voices and did nothing that would be considered abnormal. Nearly all were admitted as schizophrenic and discharged 1–7 weeks later with a diagnosis of "schizophrenia in remission"—the psychiatrists never recognized that the "patients" were totally sane and always had been. (Interestingly, many actual patients did notice that the pseudopatients were suspiciously normal.)

In another study, between 2000 and 2002, a team of researchers working for the U. S. Department of Veterans Affairs in California used unannounced standardized patients to learn how accurately physicians recorded history, physical exams, diagnoses, and treatment plans in the medical record. They sent actors to visit each of 20 physicians eight times, presenting different common complaints. The actors completed checklists of about 30 items that the physicians ought to do, each based on clinical practice guidelines and expert panels. The researchers obtained the medical records of the visits and compared them to the checklists.

The medical record did not come out looking very good. Not only did physicians fail to record 14% of what they actually did, they also regularly documented tasks they had not performed. Physicians reported that they had performed physical examination procedures, made diagnoses, and, to a lesser extent, asked about medical history and planned treatments when, in fact, they had not. That is, physicians not only did not chart everything they did, but nearly one in five things they recorded they actually had not done.[6,7,8,9,10] In another study, the same researchers demonstrated that standardized patient checklists were highly accurate when compared with covert audio recordings of the encounters. These studies established unannounced standardized patients as a "gold standard" for measuring clinical performance.

Unannounced standardized patients seemed to us the perfect strategy for studying contextual errors. But to demonstrate that doctors make contextual errors, we would need our patients to show up with problems that gave the doctors a chance to explore potential contextual complications, and we had to know that those complications, if not explored and properly addressed in the treatment plan, would result in important mistakes in care.

We came up with four basic patient presentations with relatively straightforward problems. Consider Mr. James, a 42-year-old nonsmoking man who comes to see his physician about persistent breathing problems that he believes are related to his asthma. He reports that he was diagnosed with asthma as a child but rarely had problems until about five years ago, when he began to experience more frequent occurrences of shortness of breath and wheezing. These episodes, which occur every few days, are relieved with the use of an albuterol inhaler. He and his wife now have three young children, ages 5, 3, and 2 years, who often have colds that get passed around the family. A physician recently ordered pulmonary function tests for Mr. James, which confirmed that he has asthma. Mr. James reports that he was told he would "need one of the steroid medications" and was prescribed the latest brand-name controller inhaler, which he is to use every morning and evening whether or not he is experiencing symptoms. He reports that this has helped, but that he is still periodically having problems with wheezing. A straightforward explanation for this problem is that his new inhaler is not sufficient to control his asthma. The usual solution would be either to increase the dose of steroids or to add another controller medication, such as Serevent® (salmeterol) or Singulair® (montelukast). (We mention brand names only as examples when we think they might be familiar, with the generic drug name in parentheses after the brand name. We are not recommending any particular brand of any drug.)

Our other basic patient presentations included Mrs. Collas (a 47-year-old woman preparing for hip replacement surgery who is found to have high blood pressure), Mr. Davis (a 59-year-old man with diabetes who has been feeling faint after his previous physician increased his insulin dose), and Mr. Garrison (a 72-year-old former smoker who has been losing weight). As with Mr. James, there are guidelines for each of these cases that make straightforward management recommendations if no additional information contradicts them: Mrs. Collas needs surgery postponed for a short while in order to get her blood pressure under control (possibly with medication), Mr. Davis needs to have his diet or his insulin dose modified, and Mr. Garrison needs to be evaluated for the possibility of cancer, especially lung cancer.

Next, we took those basic problems and considered two different kinds of complications. The first was a medical complication: The patient could have another disease or condition that has similar major symptoms, but that can be distinguished by additional symptoms the patient could mention during the visit. We chose complications that required the physician to make a different treatment decision than in the basic problem. For Mr. James, for example, our medical complication was acid reflux, which also can cause wheezing, but could not be treated by increasing asthma controller medications.

The second kind of complication was a contextual complication: the patient's life context could make the standard treatment for the basic problem just as wrong as it would be for a medical complication. For Mr. James, our contextual complication was that he had lost his job and health insurance, could no longer afford to pay for his controller medication, and was stretching it by using it only when he was having symptoms, rather than daily. Increasing his controller medications, and especially adding additional medications, would not help Mr. James get better.

Whenever our standardized patients acted out these cases, we trained them to offer "red flags"—clues that the situation might have a medical or contextual complication. For example, an actor playing Mr. James would always mention, "Sometimes I wake up wheezing or coughing at night" (wheezing when lying down after meals is characteristic of reflux disease), and that "Things have been tough since I lost my job."

We used what experimental researchers call a factorial design, combining the presence or absence of the two sets of complications to create four versions of each of the four patient cases (Table 2.1).

In each version, the red flags that would lead a doctor to consider possible complications were the same. But depending on the version the USP presented, the actual presence or absence of complications differed. The differences would be evident to the clinician in the responses the actor provided to appropriate questions. In other words, the standardized patient would present the same basic clues to the doctor, whether or not the version actually included either the medical or contextual complication. If the doctor explored a clue and the version included that clue's complication, the actor would respond positively and confirm additional symptoms or contextual factors. If the doctor explored a clue and the version did not include that clue's complication, the actor would deny additional symptoms or contextual factors. So Mr. James would always mention wheezing at night. In the medically complicated versions, if the physician asked for further information about that, Mr. James would reveal other symptoms of reflux, but if Mr. James was presenting a version that was not medically complicated, he would deny other symptoms (and indicate that his wheezing was not any more frequent at night than in the daytime). Mr. James would always mention losing his job, but if the physician asked about that, he would discuss losing health insurance (and

TABLE 2.1 A FACTORIAL DESIGN FOR STUDYING CONTEXTUAL ERROR WITH UNANNOUNCED STANDARDIZED PATIENTS

| | | Medical Complication (e.g., acid reflux) | |
		No	Yes
Contextual complication (e.g., job loss)	No	Basic problem	Medically complicated problem
	Yes	Contextually complicated problem	Doubly complicated problem

not taking his medication regularly) only in the contextually complicated versions. In the versions that were not contextually complicated, Mr. James would say that he was still covered under his wife's health insurance (and using his controller medications every day).[†]

To make sure that the contextual complications were just as important as the medical ones and that physicians had a fair chance of coming up with the right management plan if they knew all the facts, we presented the cases in writing to a group of 16 board-certified physicians. Each version of each case was reviewed by four physicians. In the written cases, all the facts for each case were included, and in versions with complications, the confirmation of additional symptoms was also written out. For example, in the contextually complicated versions of Mr. James, the written case included the following paragraph:

> When asked about how and when he takes his medication, Mr. James states that he is "having trouble taking his medication regularly." When this is pursued, he reveals that he does not have health insurance coverage for medication and for the last 5 years has been often unemployed. He will acknowledge that he has been using his Pulmicort Turbuhaler only when his symptoms are bad, not daily, because he cannot afford the cost.

For each of our cases, we showed that all four board-certified physicians, when given the full written case, came up with the correct management, and that the correct management was different for each version of a case.

We now had a tool that we could rely on to tell us whether physicians make important contextual errors. Everyone agreed on the right treatment for each version of each case when all the information was laid out, and that the right treatment for the basic problem would be wrong for the complicated problems. But would physicians actually seeing these patients in their offices heed the contextual clues, discover the complications, and offer their patients the right treatment for their individual needs?

[†] A video explanation of our methods, employing several of our actors role-playing both patients and doctor, is available at http://www.youtube.com/watch?v=c4pYHLtvSUg

Finally, we added one additional twist to the study design: For each script we drafted we hired two actors, one black and one white, to play identical roles. The only difference would be their skin color. This would allow us to ascertain whether a patient's race alone influences physician error-making. We had reason to believe it might, given a growing number of studies indicating that black patients get worse biomedical care. We wanted to see if these biases also increased the likelihood of contextual errors. A 2007 Harvard study, for instance, uncovered unconscious bias in the management of patients with coronary syndromes needing clot-busting drugs. Physicians were less likely to recommend these drugs when patients were black.[11]

THE DOCTOR WILL SEE YOU NOW

The Department of Veterans Affairs (VA), which runs the hospitals and clinics that provide care to veterans of the U.S. armed forces, is also an important sponsor of research on health care and healthcare delivery. We obtained a grant from the VA's Health Services Research and Development Service (popularly known as "HSR&D"), which is devoted to improving access, quality, and cost of health care. Once we had our funding, we began to work out how to send actors to doctors' offices undetected. We identified 14 clinics, some part of the VA Hospital system, some academic, some private. We contacted over a hundred physicians in these clinics and told them our plan: If they agreed to be in the study, they would have four visits from actors pretending to be patients some time during the following two years. We promised that each time they saw an actor, we would let them know as soon as they entered their note in the chart—typically within a day—so they would not need to worry when that "patient" did not follow up to receive tests they had recommended or fill prescriptions. With the help of a staff member at each clinic, we created fake patient records for each visit so our actors would see their physicians with the same kind of records that any new patient would have, including insurance or payment information. Our grant paid for the costs of the visits, so the doctors and clinics did not lose money by seeing a USP instead of a real patient.

Whenever actors visited physicians, they carried hidden audio recorders that were turned on during the entire time they were in examination rooms. We not only used these recordings to learn about what the doctors did, but also to check to be sure that the actors correctly portrayed the patient case (they almost always did). After the visit, we collected the recording, and also, with the help of our clinic staff insider, got copies of the medical record showing the doctor's diagnosis and management plan, and the bill for the visit (showing any tests or procedures ordered and conducted during the visit). All three of these—the recording, the chart, and the bill—are important to understanding what did and did not happen. The recording reveals the plan as related by doctor to patient, the chart documents what the physician claims to have observed and ordered, and the bill provides evidence of the tests and procedures the clinic believes the patient received. Only the recording is incontrovertible; physicians can (and did) mis-record in the chart, and clinics can (and did) bill incorrectly.

Before we could get started, we needed the approval of the ethics review committees at each site where we enrolled physicians. These committees, formally called Institutional Review Boards or IRBs, are an important part of research. Their job is to ensure that researchers minimize any potential harm to human research participants, that research participants are informed about what they will be asked to do, and that research participation is voluntary. Our research confused many IRBs: They were accustomed to protecting patients from physicians, but for our study they would be protecting physicians from (fake) patients. People accustomed to traditional biomedical research had trouble understanding the idea that the doctors were the subjects and the patients the observers. This confusion continued to dog us throughout the project. For instance, two years into the study, a routine audit resulted in a citation for a purported security breach. There is a rule that personal information about patients kept in hardcopy form for research purposes must be kept in a locked file cabinet in a locked office. Our fake charts were stored in an unlocked cabinet in a locked VA office. When auditors discovered the cabinet was unlocked, we explained that the records—although they looked real—contained information that was entirely fictional, and we showed them the IRB-approved protocol to prove it. They filed a citation anyway. It took numerous e-mails, phone calls, and several meetings to resolve the confusion.

Once the IRBs grasped who the subjects were, they understandably wanted to make sure that physicians' reputations would not be harmed and that they knew what they were agreeing to do in the study. IRBs look especially carefully at research that involves deception of the participants. In the Rosenhan study ("Fake Patients + Real Doctors = New Insights" section), for example, the psychiatrists never knew that they would be seeing fake patients (and did not have the option to choose not to participate). IRBs do approve research involving deception, but only when the benefits clearly outweigh the risks and no other approach could generate the needed information. Because we informed our doctors about the study and they agreed to be "tricked" into seeing a small number of fake patients, our study did not deceive the participants, and we (eventually) obtained approvals from eight IRBs overseeing research at the doctors' practices.

Our next step was to hire and train actors. We began with actors who were working as standardized patients (SP) in the Dr. Allan L. and Mary L. Graham Clinical Performance Center in our medical school at the University of Illinois at Chicago. These SPs had experience roleplaying patients to teach and test our medical students and residents. There is a big difference, however, between acting in a predictable environment like a stage or a training facility where people know you are acting, and playing a role consistently with people who have no idea you are acting. The first actor–trainer we hired performed a "dry run" at one of our VA hospitals, playing a female Air Force veteran, dressed for the part and well-prepared with a narrative about her life to tell the physician. Her boyfriend was a pilot, and she felt capable talking about flying. What she was not prepared for was the banter with real veterans that began in the waiting room:

"Hey, sister, what service were you in?"
"Ah, the Air Force."

"Really, so was I! What was your assignment?"

"I was a pilot."

"Hey, that's cool. I was a mechanic! Where were you posted?"

"Wright-Patterson."

"Really! I have a good buddy who was there probably about the same
        time as you, looking at your age. Did you know Greg James . . . .?"

"Um . . . ."

Another aspect we were unprepared for was what to do when physicians wanted to take immediate action: "I'm concerned about you. I'd
like to do blood work now . . .," "We need to get an ECG . . .," and "Please
change so that we can do a pelvic exam before you leave . . . ." USPs must
stay on script in all communication related to the research, but adapt con-
stantly to the unexpected. We developed strategies to avoid invasive procedures: "Oh, I forgot to fast for the blood test, can I come back?" "I have
a job interview and I'm running late, can we do the ECG another time?"
"I am on my cycle; we'll have to do the pelvic another day."

Our first actor–trainer decided early on that this work was not for her.
With our next hire, however, we struck gold. Amy Binns-Calvey, a professional actor, had experience as a standardized patient, a track record as
a successful playwright and producer, and, most importantly, had extensive training in improvisation. Icing on the cake: Amy's dad, at 79 years
old, was a U.S. Army veteran, lifelong actor, and theater director who also
joined our team as our oldest USP.

Preparing actors for what one of them called "doing a con" was just
like putting on a successful play and required dress rehearsals. Amy
had them practice by arranging visits to physicians who knew they were
fakes, just so the actors could experience what it was like to go undercover in the doctor's office. We discussed and planned every detail of
the process. The scripts showed the actors exactly what they had to say
and do, and where they could improvise. We created checklists to use
when we reviewed the audio recordings of visits so we would know
how well the actors kept to the scripts, and another set of checklists for
keeping track of the doctors' responses and their final care plans. Even

choosing and hiding the audio recorders was demanding. They had to be small, reliable, and acceptable to the IRBs. For example, the VA only approved one type of recorder with a special kind of encryption that its privacy rules require. Amy and the actors discussed and rehearsed strategies for hiding the devices so that they would not be discovered during an exam. Actors often hid them in a lunch bag or an eyeglass case where the healthcare staff and physician would not see them. After a few audio recorders failed or were accidentally turned off, we asked actors to carry two audio recorders—doubling the number of hiding places the actors had to find to secret the devices. Remarkably, no one's audio recorder fell out of a pocket or bag or was otherwise discovered despite hundreds of visits.

Actor anxiety diminished with experience (as did the USPs' blood pressure readings). The first few visits were like learning to drive. One source of comfort was that there was always one administrator in the practice who knew who the fake patient was. Our project manager, Gunjan Sharma, would work with that administrator to set up each actor visit, creating a fake identity in the electronic health record and, for the private facilities, fake insurance. Medical practices employed various kinds of electronic health record systems, so the procedures for creating a fake chart differed at each practice. We also needed to develop a "cleaning up" process after each visit so that any records of our USP visits were removed.

Of course, electronic health record systems are designed specifically to be secure, reliable, and incorruptible—to prevent the introduction of inaccurate data or the loss of patient records. We needed both to purposely "corrupt" each system with fake patient data and to see to it that the patient data was lost after the visit.

No health record system was as difficult to adapt for USPs as the one employed by the VA healthcare system. In a unique paradox, the VA electronic health record system is the worst for introducing fake patients precisely because it is the best for securely maintaining the records of real patients. For example, a particular challenge is that it uses veterans' social security numbers as their medical record identifiers. Creating a fake patient means adding a fake social security number into a government database. At first, we made up nine digit numbers just out of the range of real social security numbers. This worked until, by an unfortunate coincidence, the VA created filters to reject these numbers as typographical errors: If a clerk entered an out-of-range number, the system prompted the clerk to correct the error. We then went to public genealogy websites to find the social security numbers of deceased Americans and entered those. That worked until we entered numbers that had formerly belonged to veterans. The VA system keeps records of deceased veterans, and alerts a central office when anyone attempts to create duplicate numbers. Our final and most successful strategy required comparing our lists of the social security numbers of deceased Americans against a database of all deceased veterans and removing the latter from the list we used for our USPs.

We did anticipate the risk of corrupting the central VA databases with fake data; we were quite concerned about it. All information on the care of millions of veterans is stored in these databases, and researchers regularly use them to conduct studies to advance medical knowledge by, for instance, looking at whether particular treatments lead to improved patient health. If fake patient data got mingled into the central databases, it would undermine their integrity and could jeopardize future medical research. Of course, we were introducing a very small number of fake patients compared with the millions of veterans in the database, and errors are regularly introduced in real patient data simply because people are not perfect at recording medical information, but we realized that we needed to avoid contributing to the problem. We partnered with the information technology division of the VA electronic health record office. On a planned schedule, we sent them lists of our USPs' social security numbers, and they intercepted their medical records before they could be incorporated into the VA National Patient Care Database. Developing such a level of trust and partnership with VA operations was an extensive process, and we are very grateful to the people and offices who saw the value of our work for the future care of veterans and helped us overcome many barriers.

No amount of anticipatory planning could prepare our team for everything that could happen, and our actors' ingenuity and dedication was sometimes pushed to the limit. In one instance, a major storm struck at the time of a visit by a USP to a clinic. Evacuation alarms sounded, mandating that all staff and patients descend into a secure underground shelter. One of our actors was in the exam room feigning a severe degenerative condition of her hip, with a bad limp. She chose to stay in character, and allowed herself to be convinced by staff members to go to the underground shelter; accompanied by another friendly patient, she had to limp all the way down to keep up the act.

KNIGHTS IN WHITE COTTON

Imagine placing yourself in a situation where at any time over a prolonged period, you may be examined and recorded in intimate conversation with an imposter for the sole purpose of evaluating your performance at your job. Over 80% of the physicians we approached consented to participate, a testament to their bravery in being observed in a most vulnerable way. By doing so, they were putting their responsibility to patients ahead of their own comfort.

In 2008, the Council on Ethics and Judicial Affairs (CEJA) of the American Medical Association (AMA) recommended the use of "secret shoppers" under limited conditions. They wrote:

> Physicians have an ethical responsibility to engage in activities that contribute to continual improvements in patient care. One method for promoting such quality improvement is through the use of secret shopper 'patients' who have been appropriately trained to provide feedback about physician performance in the clinical setting.

The AMA House of Delegates tabled the resolution and CEJA withdrew it after a significant backlash, including concerns that it represented a failure to view the physician as a professional. Clearly, some doctors felt too threatened to endorse this new approach to observing the quality of their care, despite the suggestion that it might be a noble and ethical duty.

We reached out to friends of friends in the Chicago, Illinois and Milwaukee, Wisconsin internal medicine primary care practice community, asking them to vouch for the integrity of the research to their colleagues. We sponsored lunch meetings at every site to tell doctors about the project and address their concerns. Most signed on when we assured them that their identities would not be disclosed, that the cost of caring for fake patients would be reimbursed, and that all that was expected of them was to do what they always do—take care of people—and not think about whether they were seeing a fake patient. When physicians agreed to participate, we typically waited several months before sending the first USP, giving them plenty of time to lose interest in the study.

Once the project began, we began to collect evidence that the doctors thought they were seeing real patients. For instance, when Gunjan created the fake charts for USPs, she listed the number of a cell phone she carried as the USP's phone number. Our study called for Gunjan to notify doctors after they saw USPs, but only after the physicians' notes had been entered into the health record. On occasion, physicians were slow to write their notes, and before the note was written, they became concerned that the patient had not yet had blood drawn or other lab tests. They would then call to ask about the missing information. Gunjan, introducing herself as a wife or sister or girlfriend, provided an alibi. She might say, for instance, that her husband had run off to pick up their daughter at day care and was planning to return to the clinic lab on his day off the following week. These explanations generally satisfied the providers who were accustomed (unfortunately) to patients not following through on tests and did not suspect that it signaled they had seen a USP.

Once the doctor entered their note, Gunjan sent them an e-mail informing them that the patient was an actor. We asked them whether they had suspected that they had been caring for a USP. Many would say that, in hindsight, they had suspected it was a fake patient. But when we tried, instead, asking physicians to e-mail *us* when they thought they had seen a fake patient, we received e-mails about real patients. We expected this, because it also happened to Rosenhan during a follow-up experiment in "On being sane in insane places." Several hospitals not involved in the original study invited him to send pseudopatients to their facility, convinced that they could tell the difference between real and fake mentally ill patients. He agreed, but sent no undercover observers. All of the participating sites started reporting that they had identified the imposters—all of whom were actually real patients.

An important lesson—and an instruction we gave to all of our participating physicians—was never to assume a patient was a fake. Perhaps the only way a real patient could have been harmed in our study would have been if a doctor had called them out as fakes. The physicians were instructed never to do so, and there were no reported incidents.

Although the project moved along smoothly for the most part at the academic and private practices, we periodically lived in fear that the VA would shut the study down at VA facilities. This may seem odd, because the VA was actually funding the study. But an organization so large does not speak with one voice. The senior leadership at the time was responding to several widely publicized losses of veterans' personal information, including social security numbers, as a result of thefts of laptops and hard drives. At one VA hospital, for instance, an IT specialist lost an external hard drive containing social security numbers of about 535,000 veterans. The VA's Office of the Inspector General was omnipresent and directives to enhance data security seemed to consume the bureaucracy.

The first suggestion that authorities were concerned about our project came from Dr. Seth Eisen, the national director of Health Services Research & Development, or HSR&D, the unit that was paying for the study. He explained, apologetically, that he had been instructed to tell us we could no longer create or use fake social security numbers. This was tantamount to informing us that we would have to terminate the study. When we pointed out to him that there was no possible way that a fake patient could be harmed by disclosure of a fake social security number, Dr. Eisen agreed but said, "I think this is mainly a PR thing. The VA is just too concerned about what could come out in the press." He declined to say who was telling him we had to close shop, saying only, "They mean it."

Interestingly, after that call we never received a follow-up e-mail documenting the directive. It struck us as unusual that a senior VA official would not create the usual paper trail. Perhaps it was a friendly and informal warning, and it was up to us to decide what to do next. We decided to keep the study going.

When an e-mail did arrive, it came from the chief of staff of the Jesse Brown VA Medical Center, one of our data collection sites, with a specific order to cease the study immediately. This time we followed orders.

The VA healthcare system is divided into 21 regions, known as Veterans Integrated Service Networks, or VISNs. Jesse Brown, along with three other VA sites where we were collecting data, were all in VISN 12, which covers large sections of Michigan, Wisconsin, Illinois, and Indiana and includes dozens of clinics and seven medical centers. The Jesse Brown chief of staff explained that the request to close the study had come from the chief medical officer of VISN 12, Dr. Jeff Murawsky.

Dr. Murawsky's office, in a lovely brick building on the campus of Hines Hospital in Maywood, Illinois, about 10 miles west of downtown Chicago, had the classical feel of an admissions office at a small New England college. It seemed worlds away from the buzz and hum of the large bureaucratic institutions reporting to the VISN office. Our meeting with Dr. Murawsky also included Frances Weaver, PhD, director of the health services research center in VISN 12 and a coinvestigator on our USP study.

By a stroke of good fortune, we had a special connection to Dr. Murawsky. Several years earlier, before he had been promoted to VISN chief medical officer, Dr. Murawsky—Jeff, as we knew him—had been a primary care physician in one of the clinics where we did the early tests of methods for sending fake patients to VA facilities. Back then, we had been referred to Jeff as one of the doctors who knew the medical record system better than most and would be a good partner in the tests. We met a few times, and arranged for several actors to visit Jeff's office undercover to see what worked. As a result, Jeff understood the project and knew why it mattered.

Jeff—or rather, interim VISN chief medical officer Dr. Murawsky—was now sitting behind a desk, staring at the directive to shut down the study.

He began by asking to review each of the levels of approval we had received: Do you have all IRB approvals? Have the facility privacy officers signed off on the project? Have all your laptops and flash drives been certified as encrypted with VA-approved software? What about HIPAA authorization? (HIPAA, the federal Health Insurance Portability and Accountability Act of 1996, mandates a set of policies for protecting the privacy of individually identifiable health information during medical treatment, billing, and research.) The list went on. We had all of the documents. Jeff thought for a moment and then explained: "My job is to make sure you are compliant with all policies and practices for the administration of your duties which, in this case, is to conduct meritorious research that has been funded and vetted by the U.S. government and that meets all requirement of the VISN. You are compliant. You may proceed with the study. I'll let the chiefs of staff know."

Jeff's decision to overrule an order from a national office based on a thorough understanding of his role and a recognition that he had something of value to stand up for struck us all as brave. Not long thereafter, "Interim" was dropped from his title, and he was named the permanent VISN 12 Chief Medical Officer; a few years later, he was appointed from Washington to become VISN director. The VA is funny that way. On the one hand, it is a large impersonal bureaucracy, with countless directives rushing like rapids downhill from top leadership to individual physicians and researchers. At the same time, there is a humanistic countercurrent, with people like Jeff and Seth quietly helping small boats through turbulent water.

THE PROBLEM IS REAL

By the end of the study, our actors had made 399 visits to 111 board-certificated practicing physicians at 14 different offices. In 73% of the uncomplicated cases, physicians made the right diagnosis and ordered an appropriate plan of care (e.g., the asthma patient increased the dosage on his medication). When the actors portrayed medically complicated cases, however, the rate of success fell to 38% (the asthma patient's acid reflux was missed). But when the actors portrayed contextually compli- cated cases, the rate of success was only 22% (the asthma patient's job loss was not considered). That is, in over three quarters of cases when physi- cians saw patients with contextual factors, they made errors (Table 2.2). Physicians were more likely to discover something medically unusual about a patient than something socially unusual even when social issues accounted for the medical problems.

About half of these errors occurred because physicians failed to probe the contextual red flags. The most revealing cases in this respect are the uncomplicated cases (where probing any red flag leads the actor to deny a complication) and the doubly complicated cases (where probing any red flag leads the actor to give more evidence of the associated complication). In the uncomplicated cases, although the actors presented red flags for both medical complications and contextual complications, physicians explored the medical red flags 53% of the time, but the contextual red flags only 32% of the time. In the doubly complicated cases, where prob- ing of any kind was especially rewarded, physicians explored medical red flags 73% of the time, but contextual red flags only 63% of the time. Of course, when doctors first see a patient, they do not know how the prob- lem may or may not be complicated, so we would like them to probe all the red flags.

TABLE 2.2 FREQUENCY OF CONTEXTUAL ERROR AMONG PHYSICIANS AS MEASURED BY UNANNOUNCED STANDARDIZED PATIENTS

		Medical Complication	
		No	Yes
Contextual complication	No	Basic problem 27% errors	Medically complicated problem 62% errors
	Yes	Contextually complicated problem 78% errors	Doubly complicated problem 91% errors

We saw the same lower levels of contextual probing versus medical probing among physicians practicing in the VA healthcare system (where many patients have contextual complications and we might expect physicians to be particularly well-tuned to them) as we did in private, group, or academic practice. The difference was also the same whether the actor was black or white.

On the other hand, physicians who spent more time with patients were more likely to probe both kinds of red flags. For every additional minute of "face time"—time during the recording when the physician was actually present in the room—the odds that the physician would probe a medical red flag went up by 8%, and the odds that the physician would probe a contextual red flag went up by 5%. What this means is that for every 10 patients with contextual issues who are scheduled into 15-minute rather than 30-minute visits, one of them will present a contextual red flag that the physician will miss due to lack of time. As visits get shorter, physicians are more likely to overlook clues that may be essential to planning effective care.

Exploring alone is not enough; the doctor needs to plan an appropriate treatment. The other half of the contextual errors occurred when physicians had probed contextual red flags, but had not made treatment plans that incorporated the revealed contextual factors. In the medically complicated cases, when doctors probed and discovered medical complications, they planned the right treatment 31% of the time. In the contextually complicated cases, however, even when doctors probed and discovered contextual complications, they planned the right treatment only 20% of the time. We saw this difference in all types of practices, and for both black and white actors. Although physicians who spent more time with patients were more likely to probe red flags, more time did not lead to a greater likelihood of incorporating the results of probing into the treatment plan. Turning that around, visits in which physicians did a great job of putting together all the necessary information and planning appropriate care were not on average any longer than those in which they did not. Something about the way physicians at their best think and communicate during those visits improves care without increasing the time required to do so. We will return to this point later in the book when we discuss ways to improve contextual care.

We published the results of our study in the *Annals of Internal Medicine*, a major medical journal.[12] *Annals* accompanied the paper with an editorial by Dr. Michael LaCombe of Maine General Medical Center. Dr. LaCombe discussed more examples of contextual errors he had encountered, concluding, "How much better to learn these hard lessons from standardized patients, for both physicians and real patients, and less expensive in the long run."[13]

Media response was substantial. The study was covered by dozens of news outlets around the United States. The *Chicago Tribune* ran a front page story with the headline, "'Mystery patients' [*sic*] help to uncover medical errors," which included interviews with participating physicians.[14] One of them, Dr. Eric Christoff, generously observed "I see this as an opportunity. All of us have a lot to learn about how we can do our jobs better." We were invited onto talk radio shows to explain the study and its results.

Although we published only the formal results of the research, several unexpected observations were also quite revealing. Our actors recorded a small number of incidents that hinted at larger problems. For instance, although our black actors got the same care as their white counterparts playing the same scripts, they had a harder time signing in when they told clerks they were uninsured. They reported they were more likely to be told they could not be seen, even though they were presenting with exactly the same life story and presenting complaint as their white counterpart.

We also discovered idiosyncrasies of systems and providers that could disrupt the care or study process. Some doctors would take long personal phone calls during a visit, occasionally without even leaving the exam room. Others left the room when the patient changed, but attended to other patients, leaving the patient in a gown for extended periods of time. Some physicians focused on the computer screen, entering notes, as opposed to making eye contact with the patient. Quite a few physicians focused their attention on the weight of one of our actors, even though it was not a part of his scripted problem. He wanted to talk about his asthma; they wanted to tell him that he weighed too much and needed to diet. He confessed that he found this sufficiently irritating that it made it difficult to stay on script. Another of our USPs, after providing clues that he was seriously depressed—in accordance with his script—was told by the doctor "not to go anywhere." The doctor said he would send in a mental health professional shortly to evaluate the patient and left the exam room. No one returned in his place, and after 40 minutes, the actor left. In one private office, the physician was angry that a new patient had been added to his schedule. The USP stood there awkwardly while the physician chided his office staff, saying "you know my practice is closed to new patients." Clearly, he had forgotten about the study, and that he had agreed to the possibility of being audio-recorded. Finally, we occasionally uncovered billing problems. At one site we received a bill for electrocardiograms that our patients had declined. The clinic's financial office was skeptical when we told them these were fake patients who had refused the procedure—until we showed them the transcripts of the audio-recordings. Only then did they acknowledge that patients were getting billed as soon as a physician ordered the test, regardless of whether the test occurred. Although our focus was on contextual care, the USP process offered a much broader view of the healthcare system.

THE (ECONOMIC) COST OF CONTEXTUAL ERROR

Listening to patient context and planning the right treatment is hard. Using unannounced standardized patients, we had shown that highly skilled physicians made contextual errors frequently, both because they failed to probe contextual red flags and because they failed to apply what they had learned when they did probe. We knew from the design of the patient cases that these contextual errors would have had important health consequences had the patients been real. In health terms, these were costly errors.

Because we also obtained the billing records from the visits, we were in a position to ask whether these errors also cost more money. And because we had the medical records, we could ask another question—could we have discovered these contextual errors simply by reviewing charts, without using actors?

Calculating the full cost of medical care is surprisingly tricky. We focused on direct medical costs—how much it would cost to treat a correctly diagnosed medical problem. We also limited ourselves to costs that might be expected within 30 days of the visit. We did not try to consider indirect costs, such as the cost of transportation to the clinic or lost wages during illness, or long-term costs, such as the possibility that a patient might need hospitalization a year later. Finally, we calculated costs based on standard Medicare reimbursement schedules, rather than on the clinic's billing charges (which include overhead, profit, and other costs that are not really medical). We were being conservative: If we had considered any of these other costs, the contextual errors we found would have been even more expensive.

To calculate the financial cost of errors, we considered three different ways a treatment plan could go wrong. First, the physician might order unnecessary care that could have been avoided if context had been properly considered. This is *overuse* of medical resources. If a patient does not have reflux disease, but a doctor prescribes an antacid anyway, that is overuse. It is easy to figure out how much overuse costs—it is the cost of the unnecessary care the patient receives. When it was clear from our case that the patient would not actually receive the unnecessary treatment—for example, when the asthma patient without health insurance was prescribed a more expensive inhaler that he also could not afford—we made the conservative choice to consider the cost of overuse to be nothing.

Second, the physician might fail to order necessary care that she would have ordered if context had been properly considered. This is *underuse* of medical resources. If a patient does have reflux disease, and does not get a medication that treats it, that is underuse. It is harder to put a cost on underuse, so we made a conservative assumption. We decided that the values of common evidence-based treatments were at least as great as their costs, or else such treatments would not be recommended. So when a physician did not order a generic inhaler for an asthmatic patient, we considered the cost of that error to be the cost of the inhaler for a month.

Third, a physician might both order an unnecessary treatment and miss a necessary treatment. We call this combination of overuse and underuse *misuse* of medical resources, and we combine the cost of the overuse and underuse to get the cost of misuse.

In this study alone, we found a total of $174,000 in avoidable costs, mostly from underuse. In comparing costs of errors in different kinds of cases, we looked at the median cost of errors. The median is the value for which half of the visits with errors had higher costs of error and half had lower. We prefer the median to the more common average (the mean) because the median is less affected by a small number of extremely costly visits.

The median cost of errors in uncomplicated cases was $164 per visit when an error occurred. In biomedically complicated cases with errors, the median cost of error was $30. But in contextually complicated cases with errors, the median cost of error was $231 per visit, which is substantially higher than in either uncomplicated or biomedically complicated visits. In doubly complicated cases, the median cost of error was $224 per visit, similar to the contextually complicated cases. Contextual errors are not only more frequent than biomedical errors, but more costly when they occur (Figure 2.1). Of that $174,000 in costs of errors, almost $152,000 came from contextually or doubly complicated visits.

No more than $8,745 of the $174,000 in avoidable costs would have been detected through medical record review—these are costs of errors that physicians made in the uncomplicated cases. When a physician records a high blood pressure but fails to treat it, the error can be seen in the chart. The medical record did not help us identify contextual errors, however, because doctors cannot write what they do not observe. Even when a physician diagnoses a case incorrectly, he believes his diagnosis is correct at the time, and the treatment plan in the chart matches the (wrong) diagnosis in the chart. Physicians in our study had particular trouble identifying necessary contextual information, and so contextually complicated cases were more likely to have incorrect diagnoses and treatment plans.

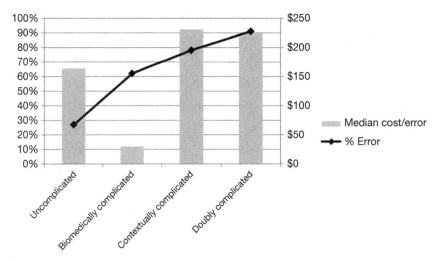

Figure 2.1
Frequency and median cost of contextual errors detected by unannounced standardized patients.

From the chart alone, however, the treatment plan is appropriate for the diagnosis, and the contextual error goes undetected. In our study, 95% of the dollar cost of error could be seen only because we had unannounced standardized patients and hidden recordings of the visits.[15]

SUMMARY

The problems we had observed with the residents proved serious and widespread among physicians in practice. As a result of our work, the largest experiment to date using unannounced standardized patients, we learned that doctors had a harder time individualizing care to their patients' contextual complications than recognizing medical complications and following guidelines. In our cases, contextual errors were more frequent and more costly than medical errors—and nearly impossible to detect without looking behind the exam room curtain and directly observing doctors caring for patients.

One thing we could not do with USPs was to find out how often real patients have the kind of contextual factors that require their doctors to learn to explore and incorporate context in order to plan appropriate treatment—that is, how often and in what form doctors make contextual errors "in the real world." To do that, we would have to watch doctors with real patients, and that was our next step.

The Problem Is Everywhere

DOCTOR: *"Do you want a shingles shot?"*
PATIENT: *"I never heard of it."*
DOCTOR: *"You didn't get any information from your friends?"*
PATIENT: *"What?"*
DOCTOR: *"Shingles! Shingles!"*
PATIENT: *"What is it?"*
DOCTOR: *"Chickenpox! It prevents you against chickenpox."*
PATIENT: *"I had chickenpox already, they say you're only supposed to get it one time."*
DOCTOR: *"Even then you can get chickenpox again, not chickenpox, it's called shingles. If you don't want it, I'm not going to force you."*

—Transcript of hidden audio-recording between
a real patient and her doctor

Studying how doctors care for actual patients may seem like a step forward from studying their interactions with simulated patients, but in some respects it was a step back. Sending physicians unannounced standardized patients is like conducting a scientific experiment in a laboratory. The doctors are the subjects and what the unannounced standardized patients are trained to say is the "stimulus." We know the cases, and what the right answers are. Nearly everything else is held constant. We say "nearly" because a working clinic is not a lab. For instance, two doctors may get the same USP, but one may be rushed at the time and the other may have no such pressure. We try to account for this difference—and any others we identify—by collecting data on whether physicians are running late when they see a USP and making allowances for that in our analysis.

When we listen to visits audio-recorded by real patients, we no longer have a say in what is going to happen during a visit and, of course, no two visits are alike. Furthermore, our strategy for measuring whether care has been contextualized also must change. Recall that we wrote the cases with USPs, so we got to decide in advance what would constitute an effective care plan for each case. We applied the validation method described in Chapter 2, in which a group of experienced physicians had to reach consensus independently about what would constitute good care for a clinical condition both with and without contextual factors noted. We cannot do that with actual patients.

So, why change our research method? First, working with unannounced standardized patients was getting to be too hard. Although the Veterans Administration (VA) had let us finish our study, it was clear we could not do anything like that again anytime soon. We continue to advocate for a simpler process and more welcoming environment for including USP research and quality improvement both within and outside of the VA. After all, nothing compares with getting accurate information about what doctors and other staff actually do in their daily work when interacting with patients. USPs are the gold standard for that.

The main reason we moved on to working with real patients, though, is that doing so addresses one big limitation of working with USPs: They tell you nothing about the diversity of challenges clinicians actually face. Our entire USP study was based on how doctors handle four common clinical situations. Of course, doctors deal with many other problems besides those four. Finally, studying contextualization of care with real patients afforded us an opportunity not available with simulated patient encounters: We could look at the impact of contextualization of care, or failure thereof, on patient health care outcomes. In other words, we could answer the question "Does any of this matter?" If patients receiving contextualized care do no better or worse than those whose care is rife with contextual errors, then who cares? Intuitively, it would seem that revising the insulin dosing schedule to accommodate a patient's new duties as a police officer on the night shift would more likely result in improved diabetes control then simply putting her on more medication. But could we show this? And, across the wide range of contextual factors that complicate patients' lives, does addressing them in care planning usually result in better health care outcomes? Only tracking the health care outcomes of real patients whose encounters have been audio-recorded and coded for contextualization of care can answer these questions (Table 3.1).

Moving to real patients required addressing several fundamental challenges. Foremost was the fact that, as far as we could tell, no one had ever asked real patients to covertly audio-record their visits with their doctors. How would patients react to being asked to do this? Second, we did not know how doctors would feel about it either. Third, after satisfying both of these stakeholders, we also would have to obtain ethical approval from an institutional review board (IRB). And, fourth, we would need a method for assessing clinician performance at contextualizing care—one

TABLE 3.1 ADVANTAGES OF STUDYING CONTEXTUALIZATION WITH UNANNOUNCED STANDARDIZED PATIENTS VERSUS REAL PATIENTS

Advantages of Using Unannounced Standardized Patients	Advantages of Using Real Patients
Control over case mix	Can measure frequency of various contextual factors
Control over contextual red flags and contextual factors	Can measure actual health outcomes and costs
Correct plan known in advance	Does not require creating fake charts, insurance records, etc.
Can be tailored to study performance in particular diseases, patient populations, etc.	Less expensive than unannounced standardized patients
Cannot interfere with actual care	

that would convincingly discern those interactions and resulting care plans that were contextualized from those that were not. We needed to develop a process that everyone—patients, physicians, and clinics—would be okay with.

Whereas in our study employing USPs we recruited attending physicians as subjects, for this project we decided to enroll resident physicians instead. This was partly a matter of convenience and circumstance. Over 100 attendings had good-naturedly participated in our research for three years, and we did not want to wear their patience thin. Another advantage of moving on to residents is that we could enroll a large number of them from just two hospital clinics that host residency training programs, instead of having to seek out attendings at over a dozen practices. The main reason, however, was that we also wanted to see whether an educational intervention could improve contextualization of care. We discuss the findings of that part of our project in Chapter 6, "Better Teaching, Better Doctors," where we explore the potential for educating clinicians to contextualize care.

Before writing the proposal we informally asked a number of residents how they would feel about being audio-recorded by their patients, if they could be assured that the data would never go to their supervisor or to anyone else outside of the research team. The most common concern raised was that they thought it would be awkward to have an audio recorder sitting there while they were interacting with a patient. When we clarified that we would ask each patient to conceal the audio recorder, they thought that was reasonable. A common refrain was, "As long as I don't need to think about it and it's not on my mind, then that's fine."

We also asked patients what they thought. (Because both these clinics are at VA facilities, the patients were all veterans.) We asked them how they would feel about collecting data using a concealed audio recorder, knowing that their physicians had agreed to participate without coercion, for a study of whether we could improve the quality of care they receive. We also explained that the data would be stored on the same secure VA server that is used to store the rest of their medical information. The main concern that came up was not wanting to risk hurting their doctors, to whom many felt loyal. Some would say, "I'm not spying on my doctor!" Most, however, said they felt fine about it as long as it could help improve care to fellow veterans.

Once we had sounded out the physicians and patients, we knew we could handle the other aspects of this project, drawing on our prior experience working with USPs. We were familiar with the various logistical challenges, legal requirements, and IRB expectations. Obtaining funding is almost always a huge hurdle, but this time we got lucky. The VA had put out a call for proposals for studies to improve care through provider education. It appeared to be one of those situations where they had some residual funds to commit before the end of the fiscal year. They wanted proposals on short notice, and said that they would attempt to fund them on the first round if possible, averting the need for resubmissions. This was in contrast to the excruciating process that typically is required. Our proposal for the USP study had taken three submissions, each requiring months of work, followed by months of waiting. This time, our proposal got approved in one cycle without much of a wait time. Like so many things in life, this had less to do with us and more to do with the context!

Once funded, the first step was to figure out who to hire for our project team. A research team typically consists of a principal investigator, coinvestigators who are career scientists or clinicians, and staff with titles such as "research assistant," "research coordinator," etc. These individuals may be aspiring medical students, professionals with a bachelor's or master's degree in a relevant discipline, or people just looking for an interesting job. They are paid from grant funding, which is inherently time-limited.

We knew two of our team would be Gunjan Sharma and Amy Binns-Calvey. Gunjan had become our expert at working with practices not only to schedule USP visits but to obtain medical records after the visit, which we knew would be just as important with real patients. Amy, of course, was our USP trainer and coordinator. Both had spent time listening to visit recordings and coding them in our USP studies, and both were eager to develop an approach to coding actual visits. We also knew, however, that we would need more people, both for coding and for recruiting patients to participate. We needed individuals who were

highly adaptive and could fulfill a variety of atypical roles requiring substantial improvisation. They would spend several days each week in noisy
clinics approaching veterans to explain our project and ask if they would
carry concealed audio recorders into their appointments. Over a period
of several years they would listen to thousands of hours of audio recordings, systematically developing a coding system under our supervision
but with much of the innovative thinking falling to them. Throughout,
they would learn the unique culture of the VA healthcare environment
and numerous complex regulations related to human subject research.

Amy, deeply involved in the Chicago acting community, introduced
us to Brendan Kelly and Naomi Ashley, both of whom had theater and
music backgrounds. Brendan was working at Chicago's Shedd Aquarium,
where he narrated the dolphin exhibit several times a day to hundreds of
screaming kids and their families. He, Amy, and a third actor also had
a long-running show called "The Weird Sisters," a wry off-color musical
comedy. Brendan proved to be highly versatile. For instance, we cast him
as the physician in an instructional video that we developed for the journal *Annals of Internal Medicine,* describing one of our studies. He looked
the part. The work at the aquarium was insecure, so Brendan was open
for a change.

Naomi is a singer–songwriter with extensive experience playing around
the city. She grew up in Nebraska and came to Chicago to pursue a career
in music. For several years, Naomi worked as assistant to the head of
the Department of Family Medicine at UIC. Naomi, Brendan, and Amy
exemplify characteristics of theater people: They are accustomed to both
highbrow and lowbrow work, to functioning in an ever-changing environment, and to living with uncertainty about what will happen next.
Actors may find themselves, in the span of a day, both applauded by well-
heeled urban professionals after playing in *Othello,* and, to make ends
meet, serving those same individuals as restaurant waitstaff. It's all in a
day's work.

But the main reason we hired Brendan and Naomi is because Amy
recommended them. Amy's signature attribute, other than accomplish-
ing so much without bothering to get a college degree (until we finally

nudged her to do so through an online correspondence program), is her exceptional judgment. If she thought a dolphin show narrator and a singer–songwriter were the right people to help us study physician decision-making, those were the people we wanted.

Once the protocol for our study was approved by the IRBs at the two facilities where we would be conducting the research, the first step was to begin the consent process, where we would obtain permission from research subjects to include them in the study. Of course, we had two different sets of subjects: doctors and patients. We started by recruiting the former. This began with our attending standing meetings of the residents, with the permission of their residency program director, to introduce them to our study. They were told that their participation would have no bearing on their status in their program. A perk, if they saw it that way, was that half of them would be randomized to participate in four hour-long workshops on contextualizing care, to occur in the mornings over several weeks in lieu of another educational conference they generally attend—and with fresh fruit and pastries from the Corner Bakery. Both those enrolling in our workshop and those in the control group would participate in an evaluation at the Clinical Performance Center with standardized patients, again accompanied by breakfast. Finally, all participating residents would be assessed from audio-recordings collected by their patients carrying concealed recorders over the coming months. No identifiable data would leave the research team. After explaining all this at resident meetings, we handed out a clipboard for them to sign their name if they were interested in learning more.

The reference to free breakfast may seem like an unnecessary detail. In our experience, however, it is just such details that make or break million-dollar studies. Getting those Corner Bakery breakfasts covered by grant money took months of paperwork and negotiation with federal budgeting and contract offices. In general, one cannot use government money to pay for food at meetings. When it became clear to us that we just were not going to have any human subjects for research unless we fed them a decent breakfast, we knew that we had to find a workaround. It turns out that if one can document that the educational sessions can only occur during times when subjects would eat, you can seek approval to find a vendor to provide food. We actually got a signed legal opinion in support of our request. The next challenge was finding approved vendors for breakfast food delivery. Although we repeatedly reference Corner Bakery above, the approved vendors would periodically change without notice. Sometimes it was Corner Bakery, sometimes Cosi or Au Bon Pain, and periodically the government would refuse to pay entirely, but we managed to use some privately donated funds to fill that gap.

Taking the clipboard of residents interested in learning more, we began to contact them to see if they formally would consent to participate. Over a 30-month period, 139 agreed to do so. Obtaining consent from our second group of subjects, actual patients, also began with asking about their interest. According to the federal HIPAA privacy law, unless a patient agrees to participate, their identity can be known only to those who are part of the process of delivering their care. For instance, the clerks who sign them in must know their identities in order to sign them in. Researchers, on the hand, may only know the identity of a patient if a patient approaches them. Hence, the patient recruitment process began when a patient approached the front desk and registered for their appointment with a clerk. The clerk was coached to mention that there was an ongoing study underway to improve care, and if the patient wished, they could help collect some of the information needed for research. The clerk would point toward a member of our team, typically Brendan or Naomi, and tell the veteran to talk with one of them if they wanted to know more.

Inviting patients to covertly audio-record their encounters with their physicians was uncharted territory. We decided early on that this had to be a soft sell. Either the veteran should be completely comfortable with the idea or should not do it at all. Many of those who said "yes" did not think it was a big deal. They casually would place the small device in a shirt pocket or bag and almost immediately forget it was there. Following the visit, if we did not spot them coming out of the office area it was sometimes necessary to chase them down the hallway to retrieve the recorder, as patients absentmindedly left with the devices in their pockets and still on. A second group of patients who also readily consented to participate harbored the idea that they were spying. Upon entering the exam room, they would take out the audio recorder, show it to the doctor and say, "Somebody out there asked me to spy on you." The residents were good-natured about it, and would typically respond with something like, "That's no problem. That's just a research study I'm in." Despite our best efforts, we could not find a way either to disabuse these veterans of their concern or even identify the concern during the consent process. Whenever they sensed any apprehension, Naomi and Brendan advised veterans not to participate. About 40% of veterans they talked with signed on.

As noted earlier, a major difference between sending in patients with narratives of our own design versus sending in real patients to audio-record encounters is that we did not even know if there would be contextual red flags to address. Whereas every one of our unannounced standardized patients (USPs) reliably dropped a clue of a possible under-lying contextual factor, such as, "Boy it's been tough since I lost my job," we had no such assurance with real patients. Health care is sometimes quite straightforward. When a patient comes in with ear pain after swim-ming in the lake during the summer, usually it is what it is. All he will need are some ear drops for presumed *otitis externa*, a painkiller, infor-mation about how to take his medicine, and instructions on what to do if things get worse. On the other hand, if the patient is hesitant about telling the doctor why the area around his ear is also black and blue, and acknowledges after questioning that somebody whacked him in the head, that's a different situation. The disconnect between the patient's story and the findings on exam is the contextual red flag that something is going on in the patient's life that is relevant to his care.

The challenge we faced was how to reliably code for the presence of con-textual red flags and clinicians' responses to them. We started by mak-ing a list of common situations that constitute potential contextual red flags, and realized several of them are evident in the medical record. For instance, loss of control of a treatable chronic condition, such as diabetes or hypertension, is a contextual red flag. If a patient's hemoglobin A1c has gone from 7 to 9 since her last visit, indicating much higher average glucose levels, that can only mean three things: either she has stopped taking her medications as directed, changed what she eats, and/or become much less active. All of these possibilities represent patient behaviors—as opposed to "under the skin" biomedical phenomena—making them contextual red flags.

Other contextual red flags identifiable just from charts include patients repeatedly missing or showing up late for appointments, or not following through on referrals they requested or to which they agreed. All these tendencies signify some sort of chaos or disruption in their lives that is impacting on their health or health care. A premise of our work is that an appropriate response to a contextual red flag is always to explore with further questioning, that is, with "contextual probing," whether there is an underlying problem that can be addressed in the care plan. Hence, if the coders agree on what is a red flag then they also agree on when probing is indicated.

When probing in response to a contextual red flag confirms the presence of an underlying problem that can be addressed in the care plan, as noted previously, we refer to that problem as a "contextual factor." In the case of patients with poorly controlled diabetes (the contextual red flag), asking them why they think their diabetes has gone out of control would constitute an appropriate probe. A response such as "It's been worse since I started working the night shift," would constitute a contextual factor that needs to be addressed in the care plan.

The final step in our coding schema, "contextualizing care," is determining whether the contextual factor, in fact, has been addressed in the care plan. For example, this might require restructuring the patient's insulin regimen to accommodate his new work schedule. In our coding, we have not attempted to second-guess what the best plan might be, only whether the plan demonstrates a good faith effort to address the underlying contextual factors that account for the contextual red flag.

In sum, our assessment process, which we call "Content Coding for Contextualization of Care," or "4C" for short, is based on tracking four elements of a clinical encounter: The presence of a contextual red flag; if present, whether it is probed; if it is, whether contextual factors are revealed; and, when they are, whether they are addressed in the care plan (Figure 3.1). Setting aside the jargon, what we are attempting to describe here is the process by which one individual considers and attends to the complex circumstances and needs in the life of another. With this basic architecture in place, the next question was whether different coders would reach the same conclusions when coding the same encounter. Such "inter-rater reliability," as it is called, is a sine qua non of any coding system.

The only way to know whether there is high inter-rater reliability is to have multiple coders listen to the same audio recording after compiling data from the same medical record and seeing whether they come to the same conclusions. Specifically, how often do different coders when assessing the same interaction agree on the presence of contextual red flags, probing of those flags, contextual factors, and whether care plans are contextualized?

Initially, the inter-rater reliability was not good. For instance, two coders would listen to the reaction of a clinician to a comment by a patient that they both concluded was a red flag, but would disagree about whether the clinician's response qualified as a probe. We faced many challenging coding dilemmas that our team extensively deliberated, sometimes for weeks. The result was a 44-page coding manual, replete with examples

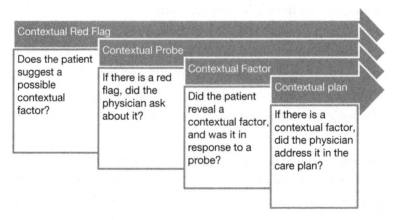

Figure 3.1
The 4C coding process.

and illustrations of every possible coding dilemma we encountered, how we decided to resolve those dilemmas, and our rationale.[1] As our four coders reached consensus on all the tough calls, and consistently adhered to the logic in the coding manual, inter-rater reliability reached an acceptable 89%. We discuss the 4C coding system in greater detail in Chapter 4.

One principle we applied across all of the tough calls was that clinicians should get the benefit of the doubt. We wanted to avoid the criticism that our coding process is a game of "gotcha!" On the contrary, we wanted a system that identified contextual errors that were hard to dispute. Hence, whenever our team reports a group of clinicians are performing poorly at contextualizing care, they have reached that conclusion using a coding system that is quite forgiving.

Once we had a system in place for determining whether care is contextualized, one methodological challenge remained: measuring the impact of contextualized care on health care outcomes. Usually, when researchers are studying how care influences patient outcomes, there is a specific outcome of interest. For instance, if a researcher wants to see whether a particular approach to counseling patients to stop smoking works, the outcome of interest is whether patients quit smoking. This is straightforward, because everyone in the study is a smoker, and the outcome of interest is always the same. In contrast, there are countless reasons why patients' care needs to be contextualized, and for each there is a different desired outcome. If a patient loses control of her diabetes, we want to see her diabetes come back under control. If another patient does not have diabetes, but keeps missing doctor's appointments for some other health condition, we want to see him making it to his appointments consistently. In short, the outcome of interest is complete or partial resolution of the contextual red flag, whatever it may be. This is the conceptual key to identifying and tracking health care outcomes associated with contextualization of care. For each red flag we would track whether the red flag resolved over time.

To avoid potential bias, we assigned this duty to members of the research team who did not have information about whether the care of the patients had been coded as contextualized or not. All they knew was the red flag.

The would know, for example, that a patient had a hemoglobin A1c of 10, signifying diabetes way out of control, but not whether the physician had identified and addressed contextual factors in the care plan. Nine months later, they would simply record whether the patient's hemoglobin A1c had gone up, gone down, or stayed the same. If it stayed the same (or went up), that would constitute a "bad" outcome, whereas any reduction in the hemoglobin A1c would constitute a "good" outcome. We would then link the two sets of data together: for each encounter, whether the care had been contextualized, and the patient's outcome nine months later.

One last point: Although our aim was to assess the "impact" of contextualization of care on health care outcomes, the study design, in fact, cannot quite do that. To prove definitively that contextualization of care causes better health care outcomes in real patients, we would need to conduct an unreasonable experiment. We would need to ask doctors to randomly provide care that is appropriately or inappropriately contextualized, and to verify that they had done so. If health care outcomes correlated with contextualization of care under these conditions, we could be pretty sure the contextualization caused the difference in outcomes. Even if it were possible for doctors to change their behaviors like this, it obviously would not be ethical for actual care. Instead, we relied on observation rather than on experiment—comparing the processes in the encounters to the eventual health outcomes for red flags in those encounters.

WHAT WE FOUND

During the subsequent months, 1,799 veterans arriving at the clinic sign-in desk were told about the study by one of the clerks. Among these, 160 were not interested in meeting with a research assistant in the waiting area, and an additional 754 declined after hearing the details of the study. We told them that we wanted to learn how doctors make recommendations when a patient's life situation is a factor in his or her care, and to see whether those doctors who had special training provided better care. Veterans learned that to participate, they would need to carry a small concealed audio recorder in their clothing or bag. We also asked for permission to examine their medical records. Finally, we reassured them that their doctor had volunteered to participate and that there was no risk to him or her by doing so.

Among those who said they would like to participate, 111 were called in to see the nurse or their doctor before we could complete the consent process and get them "wired," leaving 774 to actually make recordings. Even this group, however, got whittled down further. Although they all did their jobs, inevitable snafus occurred. There were 22 visits early on in which the recorders failed. These somewhat finicky devices had complex encryption software to meet VA security standards. There were another 32 instances in which the patient saw the "wrong" physician. This happened when doctors had others substitute for them, either because they were sick that day or too backed up with other patients. That left us with 720 recordings of visits with the correct physician.

As noted earlier, there was no way to know in advance whether contextual red flags would come up during an encounter. Once the visit was complete, and we got the recorder back, we would look for them in two ways: First one of the research team members, typically Gunjan, would review the medical record going back about a year prior to the visit to see if any from a list of contextual red flags were evident in the record itself. These had to be things that a clinician should notice and that by themselves warrant probing, such as major deterioration in a chronic condition, missing a lot of appointments, or not following through on referrals and tests. In our coding manual, we specified the threshold for each of these and we set them high. In other words, the patient had to miss a lot of appointments, or their chronic condition had to get much worse, to count as something in the chart that the doctor should not miss. Again, this was to assure that we were not accused of setting unrealistic expectations. Second, if there were no red flags in the chart, another member of the team listened to the audio recording for red flags. For instance, a patient might mention that he ran out of his meds a couple of weeks ago. Or a patient might decline a recommendation such as a flu shot, which is of likely benefit. Each of these situations suggests that something is going on in a patient's life, or that they have a particular perspective that is impacting their care, and hence, this qualifies as a contextual red flag.

For each physician, we were aiming to find the first three visits with documented contextual red flags. Because coding takes some time and we occasionally had a backlog of recordings, we sometimes collected more audio from a particular resident than we would ultimately need. As a result, in 119 instances we discarded a recording that we did not need—we already had three earlier encounters with that physician that contained documented red flags.

At the end of the data collection phase, we had a total of 601 recordings; of these, 198 contained no red flags, leaving 403 encounters in which we found at least one red flag—sometimes more. Specifically, there were a total of 548 red flags. The fact that there were only 198 recordings out of 601 that had no evidence of contextual issues that could be essential to care planning was, in and of itself, interesting to us. That was just 33%. Put another way, two thirds of encounters contained clues that something was going on in the patient's life situation that needed to be explored because of its relevance to care planning. We do not know whether that number is high or low compared to other populations of patients. (Would the medical records and audio recordings of patients from a suburban upscale community be more or less likely to reveal clues of contextual issues that are impacting on their health or health care?)

We then focused on what happened in response to these 548 red flags. First, we noted that physicians probed the red flags 32% of the time, less often than the 51% probing rate in our unannounced standardized patient (USP) study (Figure 3.2). A major difference is that in the USP study we were testing clinicians with just four cases that we had contrived. In this project, we were assessing them against "whatever walked in the door."

Second, after looking at the probing rate, we determined that in 38% of the visits a contextual factor was revealed. Although many of these were revealed in response to a probe, some were just offered up by patients, which is why the contextual factor rate was higher than the probing rate. Among the 209 contextual factors, 120 were elicited by a physician probe and 89 were revealed spontaneously by the patient. In short, some patients

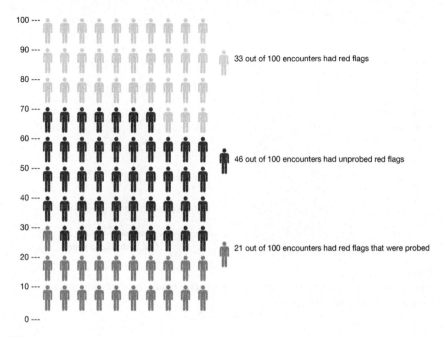

100 ---

90 --- 33 out of 100 encounters had red flags

80 ---

70 ---

60 ---

50 --- 46 out of 100 encounters had unprobed red flags

40 ---

30 ---

20 --- 21 out of 100 encounters had red flags that were probed

10 ---

0 ---

Figure 3.2
Red flags and probing per 100 real patient encounters.

fortunately will just tell their doctor what the problem is (e.g., why they keep missing appointments) even if not asked.

Third, having established the probing rate and percentage with contextual factors, we looked at what physicians did with the contextual information they either had elicited or been offered. We found that physicians addressed the contextual factor in their care plan 59% of the time, and hence, did not address it the remaining 41% of the time. This was actually better than the 22% rate for contextualizing care in the USP study. Again, it was a bit of an "apples and oranges" comparison, given that the USP study was based on just four cases. Apparently those four cases contained contextual red flags that were, on average, easier to spot but harder to address in care planning than the ones we studied in actual practice.

We learned something else of interest here. Factors initiated by probe were incorporated into the plan of care 68% of the time. On the other hand, those spontaneously revealed by the patient were incorporated into

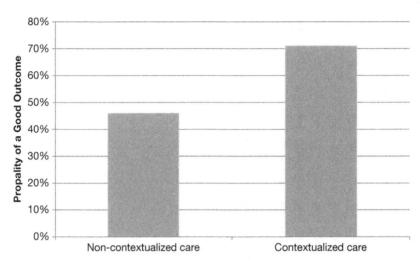

Figure 3.3
Likelihood of improved health outcomes for patients whose care was and was not contextualized by the physician.

the plan of care only 46% of the time. Doctors need to probe more, and they also need to pay closer attention to patient-revealed factors.[2]

Finally, we turned to the most important question: Are we tracking something that matters? Intuitively it seems obvious that if care is adapted to patients' needs and circumstances, they should fare better. But does our coding system of contextual red flags, probes, factors, and care plans capture the benefit we hypothesize is there? For instance, if the care plan is coded as contextualized, is the patient who has been missing appointments more likely to start making his appointments rather than continuing to miss them?

The physicians created contextualized care plans for 123 encounters and did not incorporate context into their plans for 61 encounters. Of the 123 contextual factors for which physicians made a contextualized care plan, there were 27 instances in which no outcome data were available. This occurred if the patient never returned for a follow-up visit or the outcome of interest was never documented during the nine-month period of observation. Of the 96 remaining encounters, 68 (71%) had a good outcome, while just 28 (29%) had a poor outcome. Good outcomes were more than twice as likely as poor outcomes if the clinician had contextualized the care plan. In comparison, for the 61 encounters for which physicians did not make contextualized care plans—and for which outcome data were available—just 28 (46%) had a good outcome, while 33 (54%) had a poor outcome. Good outcomes were actually less likely than poor outcomes when the clinician did not contextualize care (Figure 3.3).

In sum, problems attributable to life context were more likely to resolve in patients whose care plans were contextualized than they were to resolve for those whose care plans were not contextualized. In a statistical analysis the probability that this finding was due to chance was only 0.2%.

Substantial additional work is needed to understand how this research can change how medicine is practiced for the better. In the next chapter, we take a detailed look at how we are measuring physician performance. Subsequent chapters explore optimal strategies for using 4C to improve care.

What We Hear that
Physicians Don't

DOCTOR: *"So you quit 2011?"*
PATIENT: *"Quit smoking? It was three and a half years ago. Almost—it's
      hard when your roommates smoke . . ."*
DOCTOR: *"Any history of colon cancer?"*
      —*Transcript of hidden audio-recording between*
      a real patient and doctor

Consider the medical encounter as a conversation between a doctor and a patient who are working together to solve a problem. The physician brings to the encounter special skills and tools that may be helpful. How does the medical encounter compare with one, say, between a plumber and a homeowner? Both physician and plumber generally begin by inquiring about why they were consulted: "What seems to be the problem?" or "How can I help you today?" Typically the reply describes a familiar symptom: "I have headaches," or "My toilet is backing up." Even then, though, the astute problem solver remains inquisitive a bit longer. "Have you noticed what brings your headaches on?" or "What kind of toilet paper are you flushing down there?"

How far should the questioning go? Here is where the jobs of plumber and physician begin to diverge. When the plumber leaves, the toilet usually works and the homeowner knows to purchase a different brand of toilet paper. In contrast, physicians rarely fix a problem during a visit. If the patient came in with a headache, she will likely leave with the same symptoms. Formulating and executing a health care plan will take time, including follow-up visits. Of course, plumbers sometimes face situations like this, too, where they need to come back repeatedly to figure out what is really going on and what to do about it. In such situations, there is not much for the homeowner to do but wait for the problem to be fixed. Effective medical care, on the other hand, is rarely something that is just done to a patient. This is even true for procedures. For instance, physicians sometimes have the quick satisfaction of draining a painful abscess for immediate relief. But even then, the patient has a key role caring for the wound and following instructions about what he/she can and cannot do for a while.

In general, the problems that people bring to doctors are less discrete, and less circumscribed, than those problems homeowners ask contractors to address. In addition, in most cases the particulars of the patient matter. Oftentimes, small problems have a ripple effect. What happens if the headaches do not go away and the patient starts missing work frequently enough to risk losing a job? These second-order effects require more planning. At what point should the doctor consider adding on medications that are more effective, but also more difficult to take or riskier in terms of potential side effects? What if the patient cannot afford the medications? The circle grows ever larger.

Without boundaries to circumscribe what the doctor needs to know and consider, where does the doctor draw the line? At what point does she or he say, "That's not my problem to solve?" Years ago one of us published an essay with the title, "'I can't afford that!': dilemmas in the care of the uninsured and underinsured." The piece considered at a practical level what to do when the best care is too expensive for a patient. Should the doctor propose a less effective but more affordable alternative? Or does one recommend only the best care and leave it to the patient to figure out how to cover the cost? If the latter how far does one go in trying to help a patient obtain medications they cannot afford? Does one call the pharmaceutical company to see if they will give a discount?

When the article was under consideration for publication, a reviewer complained that it was not appropriate for doctors to get into discussions about money problems with patients. That was a matter for the financial office to handle. The doctor's job, the reviewer said, is solely to offer the best care.

But what is the "best care" when the choice is between a more effective therapy that the patient cannot afford (and ultimately might not take) and a less effective option that is within the patient's means or that he or she prefers? The answer, as we see it, is that while the first option is the better one *in general*, the latter is better *for this patient under these circumstances*. It is a physician's responsibility to draw this distinction.

An excellent plumber also adapts to the realities of a situation to solve a problem. In comparing the two occupations, however, we think the bar is higher in health care for what counts as "good enough." Whereas the plumber who finds workarounds to accommodate the homeowner's life situation is exemplary, we believe that such attention to context in medical practice is a fundamental characteristic of competence, and, indeed, of professionalism. Figuring out and doing what is best for the patient is a fiduciary responsibility. In deciding how to manage migraine headaches, including when to add additional medications, clinicians need to consider potential second- and third-order effects just to do their jobs. If the patient plans to drive across three states to drop his child off at summer camp in just a few days, might it be prudent to wait before starting him on a medication that can cause sedation, preferably until the patient has time at home to adjust to it? And if so, is it the physician's job to find out about the trip before taking out her prescription pad? The answer to both questions, we believe, is "yes."

How might one determine whether clinicians are identifying critical contextual factors, such as a patient's need to complete an imminent long car drive before starting a medication that causes drowsiness? Or realizing that a patient is already overwhelmed by the number of pills she has been asked to take and is not likely to tolerate adding one more?

In designing a system for evaluating physician attention to context, we wrestled with these questions. We concluded that although we could not comprehensively gauge how effectively doctors are contextualizing care, we could assess whether they are achieving a basic minimal standard of recognizing, exploring, and responding to clues that patient context needs to be addressed in recommendations and plans.

Hence, our approach, "Content Coding for Contextualization of Care" (4C) was designed as a measure of minimal competency. The minimally competent clinician picks up on signs that are so basic that a non-medically trained listener who is versed in 4C will recognize those indicators (what we call "contextual red flags") and formulate the questions to explore them ("contextual probes"). The minimally competent clinician upon hearing the patient's response can articulate the needs and circumstances of the patient ("contextual factors") and conceptualize how they could be addressed in a care plan (formulate a "contextualized care plan"). If our coders can do it, shouldn't we expect our physicians to do it?

The 4C system also was designed to be credible and conservative. The rules of coding need to be clear enough that different coders come to the same conclusion. In ambiguous situations, the doctor is given the benefit of the doubt. Although such a "low bar" approach does not capture many shortcomings in clinical practice, it still captures an awful lot of them. So many, in fact, that it shines a light on pervasive incompetence and identifies ample opportunity for improvement. In this chapter, we describe the nuts and bolts of 4C coding.

IS THE DOCTOR LOOKING AND LISTENING FOR SIGNS OF CONTEXT?

Because we have published an online manual on how to code using 4C,[1] we will not review that here. Rather, we would like to illustrate how 4C works, and how its design reflects a particular perspective on what competent physicians routinely should do.

Unless a patient is new to a practice, a clinician begins by looking at what is in the medical record unless, of course, the doctor knows the patient so well that she or he does not need to do so. What are the patient's medical problems? Consider, for instance, the care of a man named Don Holloway, a veteran whose diabetes control recently worsened. Mr. Holloway's hemoglobin A1c, a measure of blood sugar, has gone up to 9.8 when it used to be close to 7, an indicator that his blood sugar has been averaging way above the acceptable range. What are the trends? What has happened most recently? We think of these as first-order questions. Second-order questions go beyond the disease to consider factors in patients' lives that may be contributing to a particular clinical situation. For instance, if a chronic disease is getting worse, are there signs that the patient may not be taking medications as prescribed or following through with other efficacious treatments? For a patient such as Mr. Holloway, loss of control of diabetes is usually due to a disruption in how he is taking his medications or to his diet, although occasionally it just reflects a worsening of the underlying condition. What sort of disruptions in his life might account for the changes? The scope of questioning expands beyond the biomedical, a little like a narrowly focused lens zooming back to take in more and more of the surrounding landscape. The clue that should start this process of asking questions—the loss of control of diabetes in Mr. Holloway's case—is the contextual red flag.

When conducting our study employing 4C, we developed three levels of "contextual red flags." The first two refer to data extracted from the medical record. The difference between Levels 1 and 2 pertains to their severity. For instance, for missing appointments to qualify as a Level 1 red flag for a chronically ill patient, we decided that the patient must have had at least 16 scheduled appointments in the medical record from the prior year, and have missed at least a quarter of them. To count as a Level 2 red flag, the patient need only have missed two or more appointments in the past four months. For diabetes, the cut-off between Level 1 and 2 is a Hgb A1c of 9, so Mr. Holloway's value of 9.8 is severe enough to count as a Level 1 red flag. The distinction is useful for measuring the impact of interventions to address contextual factors. For Level 1 red flags, we measure the degree of improvement. For instance, missing only 4 appointments out of 20 in a year is measurably better than missing 8 appointments. For Level 2 red flags, we simply look for any improvement. Any improvement is scored as a "good" outcome.

One might wonder how common it is for patients to have 16 or more appointments in a year and then miss more than a quarter of them, or to take four different medications yet not refill them at least a quarter of the time, another instance of a Level 1 red flag. In fact, we found that Level 1 red flags are common. Some people get a lot of medical care, and many of them struggle to manage so much medicine and so much complexity.

If there are no contextual red flags in the medical record, the coder listens to the audio-recording of the visit for Level 3 red flags. Level 3 flags are just like Level 2 flags, except they emerge during the visit and do not appear in the medical record. In the audio of the encounter with Mr. Holloway, there were actually two Level 3 red flags: He mentioned both that he had gained a significant amount of weight since his last visit and that he had run out of a prescribed medication, an antidepressant. Upon documenting these incidentally noted red flags, the coders listened for the clinician's response to them just as they would listen to their response to Level 1 and 2 red flags.

One of the principles for deciding whether a comment during a visit counts as a contextual red flag is whether it has relevance to a medical problem. For instance, a comment by a patient that it has been tough since she lost her job is a Level 3 contextual red flag if the patient also is having trouble managing her care as reflected, for instance, in worsening blood pressure or diabetes. However, a patient's financial troubles are not relevant if they come up incidentally, and the patient is not having any trouble affording her care because she remains insured through a spouse. That is not to say that a physician should ignore such problems, only that for the purpose of 4C coding we only hold physicians accountable for contextual issues when there is an evident medical implication of not addressing them. If a patient is struggling to pay for college, that is unfortunate, but we do not see helping solve that problem as a component of the physician's job.

In the absence of Level 1–3 red flags, there is nothing to probe. If our coders have not noted any red flags, we do not expect the clinician to do so either. But if we catch a problem, we look for whether the doctor has caught it as well.

As noted in an earlier chapter, about two thirds of the encounters in our study of real patients had contextual red flags, meaning that the other third of the time we stopped coding. That does not mean there were not still opportunities for clinicians to improve the care these patients receive by getting to know their life challenges better. Rather, it meant that we did not readily identify clear-cut issues that ought to be explored by any competent physician because of their evident connection to a medical problem or health care issue.

IS THE DOCTOR EXPLORING CONTEXT?

Among those encounters with documented contextual red flags, we seek evidence that clinicians explore, or probe, them: "I see your blood pressure is out of control. Why is that?" The purpose of exploring a contextual red flag is to see if a contextual factor lurks behind it. A contextual factor is the potentially resolvable cause of a contextual red flag. Hence the best probe of a contextual red flag is one that is most likely to prompt the patient to reveal an underlying contextual factor. There are few better probes than a direct question, often beginning with "why." If someone has lost control of his blood pressure, then the doctor should ask him why he thinks he has lost control of his blood pressure. If a patient has started missing a lot of appointments, then we want to hear a question about why the patient is having trouble getting to appointments.

Our coders start by formulating what they think would be the most direct question about a contextual red flag, which we call a "model probe." Most probes begin with a summation of the problem ("Mr. Holloway, I notice that . . . .") followed by an open-ended question. After formulating a model probe in response to the red flag, the coder turns on the tape and listens for a substantively similar question from the physician. For instance, they might hear: "Mr. Holloway, I notice your diabetes has gotten out of control recently. What do you think is going on?" That counts. On the other hand, what they too often hear is: "Mr. Holloway, I notice your sugars have gotten really high recently. That could really harm you if you don't start taking your medications as you are supposed to." That statement on the part of the physician does not count. It represents a failure to explore context. It is more like a scolding.

Most of the time when physicians did not get credit for a contextual probe, it was because they did not probe at all. For instance, the doctor caring for Mr. Holloway never asked him anything that would count as a contextual probe of his loss of control of his diabetes, instead referring him to an endocrinologist. The plan reflected an assumption, likely incorrect, that the high blood sugars are due to some complex biomedical issues that require special expertise.

Although sending a patient to a specialist rather than asking the patient about what is going on is clearly a failure to probe, there were other instances in which coders heard a comment or question that seemed to fall into a gray area where it was difficult to ascertain whether the clinician was really exploring relevant context. In such cases, should the clinician get credit for probing? We developed several principles for deciding these tough calls.

First is the "Awareness Principle." Suppose the red flag is missed appointments and the model probe is, "Why have you been missing appointments recently?" Instead, the coders hear "Do you have any trouble getting to our clinic?" Although we consider that to be a leading question, and therefore, not ideal, it nonetheless implies awareness of the contextual factor, so it counts.

A second principle is to give the benefit of the doubt when it is not certain whether the provider was aware. For instance, the statement, "I haven't seen you in over a year. Can you come back next month?" does not clearly indicate awareness that the patient has been missing appointments, but it might, so it counts. Conversely, "I want you to come back next week to get your blood pressure rechecked with the nurse. Can you make it?" does not count. There just is no evidence that the doctor is aware the patient has been missing a lot of appointments.

A third principle is "Simon's rule," named after our colleague Simon Auster, who cautioned us not to assume that a direct question is always the best way to get an answer. Simon's rule says that if the patient reveals a contextual factor in response to something the physician said or asked, the physician gets credit no matter what. The concept here is that a sensitive clinician intentionally may elicit information in indirect ways, based on an intuition about how to engage the patient. And, says Simon's rule, one cannot argue with success.

Consider, for instance, a physician who says "Your diabetes is out of control," after perusing a patient's log book showing a daily record of his finger stick glucose. The comment is not even close to the model probe, "Mr. Holloway, I notice your blood sugars have been getting really high recently. Why do you think this is happening?" Ordinarily, therefore, the doctor would not get credit. In fact, the comment was not even a question. However, were the patient to respond, "Yeah, doc. I ran out of insulin. That new phone refill system is really confusing," a contextual factor was nevertheless elicited. Because the physician's comment elicited the underlying contextual factor, while also demonstrating awareness of the contextual red flag, credit is given. On the other hand, if the patient had responded with, "Yeah, I know," and the doctor asked no follow-up questions, there would be no credit for a probe.

The result of these principles is a lenient approach to coding. That is, we expect to catch all the true probes and also to count some statements as probes that might not have been. Another way to put this is to say that contextual errors are more likely than our estimates, not less.

Using these three coding principles, our team met weekly to discuss challenging situations, including any discrepancy between how two different coders coded the same encounter. Often we had what one might call "Talmudic discussions" as we parsed sentences from transcripts of audio to arrive at a consensus about how to apply the principles to ambiguous dialogue heard on audio. From these discussions, we established nine guidelines. Each of the guidelines is based on one or more of the three principles and designed to guide the coder in a particular situation.

One guideline, for instance, pertains to how one codes physicians' questions to patients that could represent either contextual probing or simply exploring the biomedical condition. Consider, for instance, the question, "Do you check your blood pressure at home?" asked of a patient with hypertension whose blood pressure is elevated. A physician might simply be trying to find out the patient's blood pressure at home. Were the patient to reply, "Naaa, I don't bother to check my blood pressure much," a physician just looking for additional blood pressure data might reply, "Too bad. It would be helpful to know what your pressures are at home." On the other hand, the physician might be asking the question to explore the patient's level of interest in, and knowledge about, properly managing his blood pressure. If this is the motive for the question, were the patient to reply, "Naaa, I don't bother to check my blood pressure much," the physician would follow up with some version of "Why not?" It is often the follow-up question by the clinician that reveals her underlying intentions—whether she is simply collecting technical details related to signs and symptoms of disease or probing patient context. Hence, the guideline: When the intent behind a probe is ambiguous, listen for the follow-up questions and code based on those.

We stopped adding new guidelines for the same reason we stopped developing principles: We did not need any more to do the job. It is possible we will need another guideline if we come across a new situation that is not already addressed with an existing guideline. The development of our coding system has been iterative.

IS THE DOCTOR MANAGING CONTEXT?

Interestingly, although the doctor caring for Mr. Holloway never probed his loss of control of his diabetes (the Level 1 red flag) he did probe one of the two Level 3 red flags: In response to Mr. Holloway's concern about weight gain, the doctor said, "Tell me about your diet and eating habits."

He did not, however, follow up on the comment about running out of a medication.

Once we have determined and documented whether the doctor is probing contextual red flags in search of underlying contextual factors, the next step is to listen for whether contextual factors are, in fact, present. Most of the time this information comes from the patient's response to a contextual probe. When asked about his weight gain, Mr. Holloway described how his dentures were no longer fitting properly and he had switched from eating fruits and vegetables to eating mostly pastas and breads, which were easier to chew. Hence, poorly fitting dentures were the factor evidently accounting for his dietary changes and resulting weight gain. Not all contextual red flags have underlying contextual factors, however. For instance, had the doctor said, "Mr. Holloway, I notice your blood sugars have been getting really high recently. Why do you think this is happening?" the patient might have come back with, "I don't know, Doc. I've been really good about taking my medicine and watching my diet." Such a response would suggest that the biochemical processes in the body that cause insulin resistance may simply be getting worse over time. Patient context would seem not to be a factor.

The second way in which coders ascertain the presence of contextual factors is by listening to whether the patient volunteers contextual information. For instance, although not asked, Mr. Holloway went on to explain why he had run out of his antidepressant, noting that his psychiatrist had left the practice and he could not get an appointment with a replacement in time to make sure he did not run out of medication. As you may recall from the prior chapter, among the encounters between real patients and their physicians in which a contextual factor was revealed, some of these were simply mentioned by patients without the physician ever asking—43% to be exact. In such instances, the physician does not get credit for probing, but the contextual factor is documented so that the coding team can see whether the clinician subsequently capitalized on the information when formulating a care plan. One striking finding that has appeared consistently in our data across several different settings is that providers are more likely to incorporate contextual factors into a care plan if they learned about them by probing rather than passively from a patient who volunteers the information.[2] This turned out not to be the case with Mr. Holloway's care, however. His physician did not address the dentures problem (which he learned about after probing) but did take care of the antidepressant problem (which he learned about despite not probing) by contacting the psychiatry clinic where Mr. Holloway receives his mental health care. This reversal of the usual pattern is likely related to lack of dental care access for veterans who do not have private coverage. (The doctor could have, however, referred Mr. Holloway to one of the free clinics outside the VA system, a list of which is in a handout available in exam rooms.) In most instances, however, it appears that doctors are more likely to follow through on contextual factors if they root out the problem themselves. If simply mentioned by the patient, the information often seems not to register.

The coding process for ascertaining whether clinicians are addressing contextual factors in their care plan follows the same strategy as for determining whether they are probing contextual red flags: It begins with the coder formulating a model response, this time for a contextualized plan of care. For instance, given that the contextual factor behind Mr. Holloway's poorly controlled diabetes is that ill-fitting dentures are interfering with his diet, the coder would craft a plan in which the clinician proposes some strategy for getting the dentures fixed or replaced. The coder would then give the clinician credit for any plan that addresses the patient's oral health needs.

The three principles—awareness, benefit-of-the-doubt, and Simon's rule—also apply to coding contextualized care planning, and many of the guidelines have analogs as well. For instance, just as Simon's rule gives a clinician credit for probing even when the clinician does not directly explore the contextual red flag but nevertheless elicits a contextual factor, so, too, we give credit for contextualizing a care plan when the contextual factor is not discussed but is addressed by the care plan. Consider, as an example, a visit at which a patient volunteers, "My meds stopped coming in the mail so I haven't been taking them." Such a comment constitutes both a contextual red flag and a contextual factor. The red flag is that the patient says he is not taking his meds. The contextual factor is the reason why, namely, that they stopped coming. Consider, now, the response: "That often happens when people don't call or come in when they run out of refills. I'll put in a new order and you can pick them up at the pharmacy. Remember to call if you start running low so we know to renew your medications." We would give full credit here for contextualizing the plan of care even though the clinician did not explore either the contextual red flag or the contextual factor.

A valid criticism of this approach could be that we are not setting the bar high enough. After all, in the example above the clinician has acted on unquestioned assumptions about why the patient is not getting his medications. What if the patient's meds stopped coming for some other reason, such as a change of address, an error in the pharmacy record regarding the correct mailing address, or someone stealing his mail? Ideally, before concluding that the patient just needs refills, the clinician would confirm whether that is, in fact, what is going on. When the medical record system is connected to the pharmacy where the patient refills his medications, such as in the Veterans Administration electronic health record, it is not hard to check. Ideally, we would like to see the clinician show more curiosity here. Figuring out why a patient's meds have stopped coming to them may involve a few follow-up questions but should not take long to sort out. Without this extra effort the care plan may simply be a solution to the wrong problem.

The reason we do not set the bar higher is that our coders have no way to ask the questions the doctor never asked, and we do not want to act on assumptions either. The physician may, after all, be correct. Hence, we give credit for any care plan as long as—implicit in the care plan—there is awareness of the contextual factor. As noted earlier, the strength of this approach is that when we do report that a high percentage of clinicians are providing care that fails to address patient context and is, therefore, not competent care, it is safe to say that we are not exaggerating. When we need a more stringent measure of skill at contextualization, we recommend unannounced standardized patients.

PUTTING IT ALL TOGETHER

It takes about one and a half times the length of an encounter to do the coding. The coders employ an algorithm that is organized according to the tasks outlined above: formulating a model probe, documenting the actual probe heard, indicating whether it was close enough to the model to count, listening for the patient to reveal a contextual factor, whether in response to a probe or unsolicited, etc. We typically audit the analysis for 10% of the encounters so that we can confirm the coder is following the coding process properly. What we want to assure is that independent coders reach the same conclusions about four data points: whether there is a contextual red flag, whether it was probed, whether a contextual factor was revealed, and whether the care plan was contextualized. In addition, for each encounter, the coder succinctly summarizes the findings. For instance, a coder might note: Patient reports weight gain (red flag); "Tell me about your diet and eating habits" (probe, awareness principle); Patient reports a high-carbohydrate diet ever since his dentures got in the way of chewing (contextual factor); No further discussion (did not provide a contextualized care plan).

This brief four-point narrative summary provides transparency. It also enables us to accumulate a growing database on the kinds of contextual issues patients face and how providers seek to address them when caring for a particular sociodemographic population. To that end, we assign each contextual factor to one of the 10 domains of context discussed earlier: access to care; social support; competing responsibilities; financial situation; relationship with healthcare providers; skills, abilities, and knowledge; emotional state; cultural perspective/spiritual beliefs; living environment; and attitude toward illness. As the data grow, with hundreds of contextual factors documented and catalogued by domain, a picture emerges of the kinds of challenges a population of patients faces. For the veterans seen at one of our sites, for instance, we see that deficits in the skills and abilities domain, such as poor vision, cognitive loss from strokes, and difficulty understanding medical information are the most common challenges. We have identified common red flags that mark the presence of those challenges. For other populations of patients, the key domain(s) of context would likely differ.

In our study on the impact of contextualization of care, we added an additional column to the spreadsheet: red flag outcomes. A good outcome is defined by an improvement over time in the original red flag(s), such as weight loss or access to psychiatric medication, in Mr. Holloway's case. A poor outcome is no improvement or worsening of the red flag(s). As detailed above, for Level 1 red flags we also measured incremental improvement. Missing four appointments instead of eight in a comparable period of time would be considered an improvement.

We only track contextual red flag outcomes for encounters with an identified contextual factor. Hence, Mr. Holloway's Hgb A1c would not count because it was never probed and no contextual factor was explicitly revealed. We say "explicitly" because it may well have been the same factor linked to his weight gain, those ill-fitting dentures.

In order to avoid bias, we track outcomes without knowing whether the care plan was contextualized or not. Hence, a coder designated to follow up on each patient nine months after their visit to see what happened with the original contextual red flag will not know whether the care plan addressed the underlying contextual factors thought to account for the red flag in the first place.

USING 4C TO ANSWER TOUGH QUESTIONS

Inattention to context, and the resulting contextual error, may simply reflect the limitations that the individuals functioning as clinicians bring to the workplace. Regardless, we have no reason to believe that those limitations are irremediable. These same healthcare professionals have the skill and intelligence to detect subtle physical findings or changes in laboratory values to recognize biomedical disease. They are smart. They chose a healing profession and care about patients as a group. It seems unlikely that when they overlook the comment, "Boy, it's been tough since I lost my job," it is because they are either unmotivated or incapable of recognizing why such a comment may be relevant to the care of a patient who has been prescribed a medication they cannot afford. In the next chapter, we explore why clinicians with extensive education and obvious intelligence perform so poorly outside of the biomedical sphere.

PART II

Solutions

Causes

"I'm the doctor, not the other way around."

—Comment by a physician who repeatedly misses patient context

Our system, "Content Coding for Contextualization of Care" (4C), is a process for determining whether a particular care plan is contextualized. But we want to know more. We want to know what physicians who contextualize care do that other physicians do not. What is different about a doctor who responds to the comment, "Boy, it's been tough since I've lost my job," with "Sorry to hear that. It's a tough economy. Do you have any allergies?" and a doctor who responds with, "Sorry to hear that. What are some of the challenges you are facing?"

To explore this question we went back to the audiotapes from the unannounced standardized patient (USP) study. The value of those tapes, as noted earlier, is that they enable head-to-head comparison of physicians with the same "patient." As you will recall, there were four different patient narratives, each with four variants: baseline, biomedically complex, contextually complex, or both biomedically and contextually complex. We compared five low-, five medium-, and five high-performing physicians from that study. Their performance rating was based on how well they did in each of their encounters. A physician was classified as a low performer if he or she never probed contextual issues in any encounter. A medium performer probed contextual issues on at least three out of the four encounters, but she or he neglected to create a contextualized care plan in the two variants where there were contextual factors to address, that is, in the contextually complex and the biomedically/contextually complex variants. A high performer not only probed contextual issues on at least three out of the four encounters, but also formulated a contextualized care plan in at least one of the two contextual variants. In short, low performers were those who were oblivious to context; medium performers notice and explore context, but do not use what they learn; and high performers formulate contextualized care plans. The term "medium performer" is perhaps a misnomer, given that—as with the low performers—when context matters, patients of these physicians leave with the wrong care plan.

With 58 audio recordings of these physicians (two of them had only three recordings each), we asked the question: How do these three groups of doctors differ in how they reason through clinical problems, as reflected in the ways in which they communicate with their patients and plan care?

Asking how doctors contextualize care is quite a different question than asking whether or how frequently they do so. In contrast to a deductive approach, where we start with a supposition or theory of what is going on and then test it, inductive exploration is about starting with what we observe and formulating theories. Theories are formulated from data, ideally without presupposition. After watching a process closely and repeatedly, from various angles, at a certain point one says, "I think I know what is going on here." That is a theory. We continue to observe for a while longer, perhaps making adjustments to our theory along the way, until we realize that there is little to gain from further observation; we are acquiring no new insights, just further evidence that our theory explains what we are observing. Qualitative methodologists call this point of arrival "saturation."

Several members of our research team, together with Dr. Carol Kamin, a medical education researcher experienced in analyzing qualitative data, independently listened to the audio recordings, knowing in which group—low, medium, or high performing—the clinician had been placed. Early on they listened repeatedly to a sampling of audios from each of the three groups to catalog every discernible communication behavior. The list of over 80 behaviors includes "engaging in small talk," "asking permission," "veering off topic," "addressing patient's concern," "encouraging," "using medical jargon," "typing while patient is talking," "interrupting," "scare tactics," etc. Once they reached saturation, they agreed they could continue to add to the list if any new behaviors were heard on subsequent tapes.

Cataloguing communication behaviors is not new. The best-known typology designed specifically for clinician–patient interaction analysis is the Roter interaction analysis system, or RIAS, named after the pioneering Professor Deborah Roter at Johns Hopkins University. RIAS is much more sophisticated than the list we developed. It has been extensively refined as a methodology for coding every utterance between a physician and patient into a mutually exclusive category. Hundreds of studies and papers utilize RIAS to parse conversations in the doctor's office, so that those conversations can be analyzed to address research questions.

Our research team has substantial experience with RIAS. When we conducted the original USP study, our grant hired Dr. Roter's group to conduct an RIAS analysis of all 400 audio recordings. We were provided with a massive spreadsheet in which every utterance of every encounter was assigned to a particular communication behavior interaction type. We then looked to see if any of the communication behaviors were associated, either independently or clustered together, with contextualizing care or with failure to do so. The only (weak) association was with "backchanneling." Backchanneling is based on the linguistic concept that in a conversation, at any one time, one person is generating the predominant channel and the other person, through vocalizations like "uh-huh" and "sure," is sending messages as well through a backchannel. If this connection is real, it suggests that physicians who do a lot of affirming vocalizations also are more likely to contextualize care. It is an interesting association but clearly not a strategy for evaluating whether doctors are contextualizing care.

It was the absence of such a strategy, in part, that led us to develop 4C. Conceptually, the difference between RIAS and 4C is that the former codes for process and the latter for content, hence the name "Content Coding for Contextualization of Care." Consider, again, our "patient" who said, "Boy, it's been tough since I've lost my job." In the first instance, when the doctor replied "Sorry to hear that. It's a tough economy. Do you have any allergies?" RIAS coded the first utterance as "empathic socio-emotional exchange," and the second utterance about a tough economy as "legitimizing." 4C codes the exchange as a failure to probe a contextual red flag. In the second instance, the doctor asks "What are some of the challenges you are facing?" and the patient acknowledges that he is having trouble paying for his asthma medication. The doctor switches him to a lower-cost generic, noting that it works just as well. RIAS codes the doctor's question as "open-ended psychosocial questioning," and the instructions to switch medications as "task focused biomedical information giving." These utterances are then grouped into a ratio with utterances that are considered to be "patient-centered," such as psychosocial questioning in the numerator, and those considered "doctor-centered," such as biomedical questions in the denominator. RIAS codes the second example as less patient-centered than the first based on a formula, and 4C codes the second example as probing context and contextualizing the care plan.

As these examples illustrate, RIAS is focused on each discrete utterance rather than the logic of the exchange. A physician is coded as more patient-centered for empathic utterances and less so for issuing directives, even when in the first instance she entirely overlooks the patient's problem and in the latter plans a solution. Content coding is just what it sounds like: listening to and processing the actual content of an interaction. RIAS does not concern itself with the logic of an exchange. Each utterance is coded in isolation.

Interaction analysis is useful to the extent that the process and content of human communication are related. It is a proxy measure for what is really going on. For instance, people who ask a lot of open-ended questions in an interaction are likely learning quite a bit more than others who are doing most of the talking while in a similar role. RIAS would code a physician who is asking a lot of open-ended questions as more attentive to the patient's needs than one who is not. In most, but not all instances, that may be the case. But not always. For instance, one of our actors happened to be overweight, although his weight had no bearing on his reasons for visiting a doctor. Several doctors asked repeated questions about how he planned to shed some pounds, but none about the contextual red flags related to his inability to afford needed medications. The actor would tell them he was not interested in losing weight, but they would keep coming back to it. Based on RIAS coding, the open-ended questions would count toward patient-centeredness even though the patient's stated preferences are ignored. Hence, without any knowledge of the content of the interaction, one can draw unreliable inferences about whether care is, in fact, centered on the patient's needs and circumstances, or context.

RIAS analysis does not correlate with physician attention to contextual issues because it is based on analysis of short snippets of speech, each in isolation. As our research team compiled their own list of communication behaviors, they were mindful of this limitation. Clearly, identifying the differences between physicians who think contextually and those who do not requires more than cataloging differences in types of utterances. "Simon's rule," for instance, described in the previous chapter, accommodates the differences in how clinicians may communicate to achieve the same end. Simon's rule gives the clinician credit for probing for context if something she said in lieu of a question prompted the patient to reveal a contextual factor.

Hence, our effort to create our own list of interactional behaviors and then document the presence or absence of those behaviors was only a means to an end, not an end in itself. The purpose was to engage the research team deeply and rigorously with each recording in a manner that diminished preconceptions and facilitated making comparisons. The goal was to look for broader patterns of interaction—rather than just clusters of utterances—that differentiate physicians across the three groups.

When one lines up our list next to Roter's, the differences are evident. Hers is a well-organized typology designed to have universal application for coding physician–patient interaction. Ours, in contrast, is just a long list of interactional idiosyncrasies that we have noticed while conducting our particular analysis. "Veering off topic," for instance, is a behavior we heard among physicians who are most often inattentive to context. But it is not an RIAS code, probably because it requires attention to content. One cannot know whether someone is veering off topic unless one knows when they are on topic.

The list of behaviors assembled by our team was compiled using software designed specifically for content coding. Content analysis software is basically a technological alternative to the stack of index cards once so common in college when writing research papers. In the old way, insights and the evidence to back them, with the source title and page numbers noted, were scribbled on cards. The cards were then laid out on a large table and shuffled around until patterns were noted and the thesis for a term paper hopefully, eventually, with enough hot coffee, came into focus. Content analysis software not only reduces the surface area needed for this work, but amplifies one's capacity to identify, organize, and analyze patterns in text or on audio.

There are several such programs, and we used one called NVivo, which calls each behavior a "node." NVivo is designed to facilitate the approach we adopted.[1] Once we had a nearly exhaustive list of nodes, the team members worked their way through transcripts of all the recordings, assigning nodes along the way. They listened to the audio in batches, grouped according to the physicians' performance, while fully aware of the performance group to which that they were listening. This "nonblinded" method is typical of qualitative analysis. First, one listens to either all of the high or low performers, both to assign nodes and to discern overarching patterns of communication. Then one does the same with those in the contrasting group. One compares and contrasts until one is convinced that any distinguishing patterns one detects are really there. Finally, we listen to recordings in the middle to see if they fall along a spectrum, with characteristics of both high and low performers.

Although each member of the research team did this work independently, they conferred whenever one of them heard a new node. If one noted a theme that the others had not, everyone would go back and listen again. This did not happen often, because most behaviors were assigned a node in the first phase of the study. Gradually, the preliminary list became all-inclusive, in other words, fully saturated.

Over time, consensus developed around six axes that differentiate physicians who contextualize care from those who do not. Each axis runs along a continuum between opposite poles—adjectives or behaviors—that differentiates noncontextualizers from contextualizers.

The first axis extends between rigid and flexible approaches to communicating with patients about their health needs. Noncontextualizers are the rigid ones, controlling the pace and content of the interaction without accommodating input from the patient. At the extreme end of the spectrum, physicians are heard plowing through the visit, pushing whatever the patient says off to the side. Such encounters have a forceful, distorted quality, making them hard to follow as illustrated here:

> DOCTOR: "Have you ever had a PFT done?"
> PATIENT: "No, um, I've never blown into a machine. I have a . . ."
> DOCTOR (interrupting): "Albuterol, no the spirometry?"
> PATIENT: "No, the . . ."
> DOCTOR: (interrupting): "Spirometry, spirometry done, did you blow into a line?"
> PATIENT: "No, all I have is . . . what do you call it? The peak flow meter."

Even an experienced primary care physician has trouble making sense of such a fragmented conversation. PFT refers to "pulmonary function test," which involves blowing into tubes connected to a computer that measures lung performance, a process termed "spirometry." It appears from the patient's statement, "I've never blown into a machine . . . " that he actually understands the question. Before he gets cut off, he is trying to explain that while he has not had PFTs, he does use another machine at home to check his airflow, namely, a peak flow meter. The physician is too impatient to allow him to complete the sentence and incorrectly assumes the patient is about to tell him he has a home nebulizer, which is a machine used to blow albuterol, an asthma medication, into the lungs. His interruption with, "Albuterol, no the spirometry?" seems to be shorthand for "I know you are about to tell me that you have an albuterol machine, but that's not what I'm asking. I'm asking if you have had PFTs?" If he had not interrupted, he would have learned that the patient did understand the question—as soon becomes evident. To further complicate matters, when the patient tries again to explain that he does understand the question, beginning with "No, the ... ," he is cut off again. Then the whole crazy inter-rogation begins all over again with the physician practically crying out "spirometry, spirometry ... did you blow into a line?" to which the patient is finally able to answer, "No, all I have is ... the peak flow meter." The telegraphic dialogue has the feel of two people who have fallen overboard and are grappling for a lifeboat. One screeches orders or questions at the other, then becomes too impatient to await the reply before starting over again. While the physician is talking, one hears the clatter of his typing on a keyboard, almost as if there is a third party taking notes.

This rigid highly directive approach is invariably accompanied by a unilateral decision-making style. The physician follows the above with, "I will give you albuterol; and we don't have Pulmicort, we have some other kind." To the uninitiated it sounds like he is saying "I will give you alb-uterol because we don't have Pulmicort ..." In fact, these are two differ-ent classes of medication often taken together. What he means is, he will renew the albuterol metered dose inhaler (MDI) prescription (not to be confused with albuterol nebulized, which the patient does not take), and substitute some other comparable medication for the Pulmicort, which the patient is also taking. The physician then says that he is sending the patient for "blood work," without seeking his permission or providing an explanation. The possibility that the patient may not be able to afford the test or medication is never considered, despite statements the patient makes earlier in the visit about being recently unemployed.

These types of interactions are characterized by the physician having an agenda, and the patient's input not deterring the physician from that agenda. The physician is the boss. He is not listening because he thinks he already knows what needs to be done. He is oblivious to context.

Contrast such an approach with one that is more flexible and open to input from the patient. These interactions feel more relaxed. The physician's questions are most often open-ended, and she or he allows the patient to complete a response. The doctor pays attention to what the patient is saying, asking a lot of follow-up, clarifying questions. There is a balanced back-and-forth aspect—this is a real conversation. The sound of typing in the background is absent during conversation. The interactions usually begin with a greeting followed by getting down to business, but with the patient setting the agenda:

DOCTOR: "So, what can I do for you today?"
PATIENT: "I'm thinking of getting hip surgery. When I saw the hip doctor my blood pressure was high. I haven't seen a general doctor in a while, so I thought I'd get that checked out, but it was good today, so I had a couple of other questions."
DOCTOR: "Alright, sure."

It's not that physicians do not have an agenda during these types of interactions. You do hear them working their way through topics they want to cover. But there is a flexibility, a willingness to digress as needed before returning to their mental map. In the above example, the physician responded to the patient's concerns before more history taking. Doctors with a flexible approach open the doors to hearing context, talking about it, and addressing what they learn in the care plan. A remarkable, and counterintuitive finding mentioned earlier, is that these visits do not take any more time. Although they are superficially more leisurely, the approach is, in fact, more focused. It is just that the focus is on the patient rather than on the physician's to-do list. Figuring out what is really going on with the patient is often an efficient means to a logical care plan, because such an approach uncovers the actual underlying issues that account for the presenting problem.

Once our team came to a consensus about the characteristics of rigid versus flexible interactions, two members of the team, Amy and Gunjan, listened to all 15 physicians and assigned them a score from 1 to 10, with

10 signifying the most flexible. The score assigned each physician was based on listening to their four encounters (just 3 encounters for two physicians, as noted earlier). The concept, here, is "rigidity in interactions" and the connotative (nonliteral) meaning of it is hard to define. It is evident, however, in the high degree of concordance among the research team members listening to the audios as to where on the scale a particular physician belonged. Furthermore, the raters' scores correlated with physicians' performance at contextualizing care. The doctors who got a high score for flexibility, such as an 8, were most likely to contextualize care, while those who received a 2, for example, were among the least likely to perform well. We used the same scale for all six axes, with a high score indicating more of the trait associated with high performance at contextualizing care.

In addition to assigning scores, the investigators took notes independently, explaining why they assigned a particular score and providing examples from each audio. For instance, after listening to all encounters with a particular physician designated in our database as Dr. A., both raters assigned a score of 2 for flexibility, and one of them wrote: "This doctor generally launches right into providing education, ordering general screening and tests, never seeming to register that the patient may be there with a specific concern. He never asked questions. It seemed as though he just assumed the patient was there for general care. He never asked, 'Why are you here?' or anything like that. He frequently refers to himself in the third person as in, 'We as internists . . .', or 'We as doctors . . .'"

In several encounters, the patient had difficulty mentioning the contextual red flags, because he would get interrupted, typically by Dr. A. finishing the sentence for him, but not in the way the patient had intended. In other respects the doctor seemed quite supportive. He was reassuring, encouraging, and provided a lot of instruction. Typically, when the patient brought up a contextual issue, the doctor would say, "We will talk about that," but would never return to the issue.

The other rater echoed these observations. She writes that "He (Dr. A.) loves to tell patients what internists do for patients in general with such conditions," "doesn't let patients finish what they are saying," and "explains medical conditions very nicely." Overall, one has the sense of a physician who energetically pursues his role as he sees it, that is, as an authoritative lecturer who speaks for his profession to an audience of one. He will not be derailed by pesky questions or concerns patients raise about the struggles in their lives. During the encounter in which a woman comes in requesting a preoperative evaluation for hip surgery and mentions that she is caring for her ill son, he mutters, "That's something we'll have to come back to," and continues down a checklist of preoperative testing questions. He never comes back to it. The physician is "rigid" in the sense that he cannot adapt to the situation as it evolves. He is unable to bend away from his trajectory even when prompted to do so.

In contrast, the five physicians we studied who were all successful at contextualizing care were far more willing to go off track as issues arose. Consider physician Dr. L., who received scores of 8 and 9 for flexibility from the two independent raters. One rater writes, "this doctor starts by exploring the complaint—and spends time clarifying, not stopping at just one detail from the patient about her life situation ... then, he states, 'let's take a break to go over your history' and he reviews what he's heard, saying 'you can tell where I'm going.'" The other rater, listening to the same encounter, writes, "he catches the contextual red flag the moment the patient brings it up." Listening to another audio of the same physician, in which a patient reveals that his daughter died in a domestic violence incident, the same rater notes how the doctor's openness to take it all in and respond to what he hears is a flexibility that reflects thinking contextually. She highlights a specific comment by the physician to the patient: "It's hard to ignore the fact that there's a lot of stuff that's happened to you over the last year. Do you see what I'm saying, the weight loss, your daughter obviously, the job, you know, so a lot of things have changed that might be influencing what's going on with your initial concern here with the weight loss." Other physicians, those with low scores for flexibility, did not seem to have trouble ignoring such facts.

The second axis to emerge was a "systems reviewing versus theory building" approach to history taking. "Systems" doctors seemingly structure each visit around a list of questions that they follow. The questions may be memorized or written out and kept on hand. The approach reflects a traditional method for training second-year medical school students in which trainees are taught to work their way through a standard list of questions known as the "review of systems," or "ROS." The "systems" in ROS refers to organ systems, such as the cardiovascular system (CV) or the gastroenterological system (GI). A review of the GI system would include questions such as, "Are you having any diarrhea, constipation, heartburn, gas, etc . . .?" Because the questions are intended to be addressed to patients, lay terms are used (e.g., "gas" instead of flatulence or "heartburn" instead of "gastroesophageal reflux").

A rote, standardized approach encourages thoroughness and precision, even down to what words to use when asking questions. The ROS is just one component of the medical encounter that is taught and learned this way. Medical students are generally taught a routinized approach to the physical exam, often conducted from head to toe. Once they become more advanced, they are not expected to carry out every step every time, but rather to exercise judgment about what to ask and what to examine. The point, however, is that they begin with a comprehensive foundation built on structure and habit.

Learning to do things by following a sequence also has its place in professional practice. In his book, *The Checklist Manifesto: How to Get Things Right*, Atul Gawande documents how checklists can save lives both in and outside of health care by assuring that effective processes are correctly carried out.[2] Checklists help pilots, doctors, and anyone else doing tasks with many difficult-to-remember steps that must be meticulously followed. Checklists are critical in the operating room or intensive care unit where missing a step in a series of tasks can be disastrous.

But there is an important distinction between learning a series of steps for routinizing critical practices and doing so for building a foundation of knowledge. In the former case, it is critical to follow the checklist every time; in the latter, we hope that the learners will grow beyond the foundational checklist. Each has its place. In practice, checklists keep the mind from drifting away from what needs to be done when what needs to be done is always the same. But in education, they provide a foundation upon which the mind can apply higher order cognitive skills to address unique situations.

Exercising higher order cognitive skills—also referred to as "critical thinking"—is a key goal of medical education. In the 1950s and 1960s, educational psychologist Benjamin Bloom developed a taxonomy of learning objectives, which includes six levels of learning in the cognitive domain (Figure 5.1).[3] The lowest level, rote memorization, includes knowing terms, facts, or the sequence of a process. The second level is "comprehension," which is demonstrated by explaining what the memorized information means or what it is for. The third level is "application," which is demonstrated when the information is used as intended to accomplish something or solve a problem.

For processes that need to be done the same way over and over again, this is as high as you go in Bloom's taxonomy. Correctly applying information to complete a task in the right sequence at the right time is the goal. But for processes that need to be individualized, that is, contextualized, three higher-order critical thinking skills are variously required: analysis, evaluation, and synthesis—the latter also termed "creation," given that it generates a new coherent whole picture of a situation. This is what we mean by "theory building." The requisite cognitive skills are at the top of Bloom's taxonomy. When we talk about learners lacking critical thinking capacity, we are describing the top half of Bloom's hierarchy as missing.

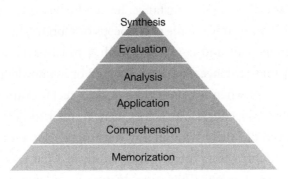

Figure 5.1
Bloom's Taxonomy.

Critical thinking is what enables us to recognize, for instance, a discrepancy between what we are told and what we observe. A patient tells us they are doing fine, but we notice that they are losing control of their health, as reflected in rising blood sugars and blood pressure. Critical thinking also is evident when we combine data sources to arrive at new insights, as when we note that an elderly patient who has been losing weight and is scheduled for an extensive series of tests to look for a hidden cancer may have social reasons for weight loss in light of evidence that he is carrying around bedding and mentions sleeping in a friend's basement. As a theory emerges about the possible reasons for the weight loss, the clinician who is thinking critically will evaluate the situation by formulating appropriate questions. Higher order thinking and the questions it generates lead to a new plan that incorporates complexity.

Exemplifying a systems reviewing rather than a theory building approach is physician Dr. N., who launches into a checklist of closed questions without asking a patient why he has come for an appointment. When the patient exhibits repeated confusion about medication and dosages, the physician simply keeps correcting him rather than noting the confusion as a new problem. When the patient mentions struggling to care for a parent with Alzheimer's disease the physician ignores the comment, presumably because it is not germane to the list of questions he wants answered. This doctor is obviously also rigid, by the way.

This same physician, like others who are inattentive to data that is not a response to their prescribed questions, also seems detached from his patient as a social being. For instance, he can be heard typing throughout the interview. And when his pager beeps or vibrates, he can be heard making a phone call and conversing with a third party, all while the patient is in mid-sentence—with no apology or acknowledgment of an interruption. And when it comes time to do a rectal exam and to have an EKG—both procedures our actors were trained to decline—he just went ahead and did them without any warning, explanation, or seeking of permission. Our actors literally did not know what was about to hit them until it was too late. This same doctor also attempted humor disconnected from the patient's reality, at one point asking, "Why did you survive Vietnam?" In a population of individuals struggling with post-traumatic stress disorder (PTSD) and survivor's guilt, such a comment may cause incalculable harm. This provider, who received a score of 1 out of 10 for a theory building orientation, missed all contextual red flags that were presented to him. But he got through his checklist.

At the other end of the spectrum were three clinicians who received an 8 out of 10 for their theory building approach when new data were dangled in front of them by one of our USPs. Physician Dr. V. is the prototype, persistently following up questions and chasing leads to arrive at a new understanding of a problem. For instance, in the case of the patient who has lost control of his diabetes, the physician first asks about how the patient is taking his insulin, and then keeps asking questions until the story tumbles out: The patient has trouble keeping track of his meds because of a learning disability; that until recently he had help from a friend and neighbor; and that he lost that support when he moved to town to help care for a parent with dementia. The clinician then arranges for the patient to meet with a nurse educator who specializes in diabetes education.

There are considerable similarities between the first two axes: the theory building doctors are also the flexible ones, and the systems obsessed doctors are also rigid. The terms simply reference different manifestations of their behaviors. In the former, the flexibility is demonstrated by an inclination to keep the conversation open-ended—to let it go where the patient wants it to go. The theory building inclination is demonstrated when, following a red flag, the clinician starts to ask sequential targeted questions that home in on the underlying issues that account for the red flag. Conversely, in the latter, rigidity is demonstrated by an inclination to herd patients through the interview, seeing the particulars of their situation, when they emerge, as a distraction from the task at hand. When these doctors adhere to a systems approach where the interview must follow the clinician's checklist, this is just one particularly scripted version of rigidity.

The third axis could be described as extending from premature closure to open-mindedness. If a patient comes in with headaches, and they have a history of getting sinus headaches during allergy season, and it is allergy season, they probably have sinus headaches due to a seasonal allergic reaction. Right? But, if that is the case, then why are they coming to see the doctor? Wouldn't they be the first to recognize the pattern? Hence, the red flag is that they are seeking medical care for a condition with which they are already familiar. Premature closure is a type of cognitive error that has been written about quite extensively in the field of medical decision-making.[4] It occurs when clinicians reach an incorrect conclusion early on in the visit about what they believe is going on—typically based on pattern recognition. Premature closure can lead to an incorrect medical diagnosis when a clinician misses unusual signs or symptoms of an uncommon condition because the rest of the clinical picture points to a common condition. It leads to a contextual error when the clinician misses contextual red flags. Showing up in the doctor's office for a problem the patient is probably familiar with and knows how to handle on his or her own is a contextual red flag. The astute physician will ask whether anything is different that prompted the patient to seek medical attention. Hence, open-mindedness can prevent missing both biomedical (e.g., brain tumor) and contextual factors (e.g., domestic violence) that would otherwise not emerge because the clinician already has decided he or she knows what the problem is.

When a patient with diabetes complains of episodes of nearly passing out, and says they feel better after they eat something or suck on a candy, that is a sure sign their blood sugar is getting too low (i.e., they are getting hypoglycemic). Hypoglycemia is dangerous and will prompt physicians, when they hear about it, to reduce the insulin dosage a patient is taking. In our USP case, the actor role-played a patient who was so confused about his insulin dosing because of a learning disability that he simply was not able to follow the directions without the assistance he had received from his friend and neighbor prior to a recent move. Physicians who had predetermined that they needed to adjust his insulin dosage asked a lot of closed questions, missing the larger issue and the numerous hints that there was a cognitive challenge they needed to address:

DOCTOR: "All right, so you are on Lantus" [a brand name for a long-acting form of insulin]?

PATIENT: "Lantus, yeah."

DOCTOR: "How much Lantus do you take?"

PATIENT: "Uh, I get the numbers mixed up, and that's the problem."

DOCTOR: "Lantus is a once-a-day bedtime."

PATIENT: "Are you sure?"

DOCTOR: "Right."

PATIENT: "Just once a day? Uh, that's 24 units, and um, Novo .... Nova? Novalog? [a short-acting insulin]

DOCTOR: "Mmm, mmm, Novolog, the super fast-acting one."

PATIENT: "Right."

DOCTOR: "And how many units of that do you take?"

PATIENT: "Uh, uh, I take 12 units of this . . ."

DOCTOR: "Before each meal or what?"

PATIENT: "With each meal."

This exchange, and others like it, would drag on until the doctor had made a decision about what dosage adjustments to make, and would tell the patient what to do. The patient's confusion was treated as a distraction because the clinician already had decided that the problem was that the patient was on too high a dose of medication, and it was just a matter of figuring out what changes were needed.

Contrast this mindset with that of clinician Dr. V. described above, who quickly elicited the narrative that the patient was unable to keep track of his medications since losing the support system that he had had in place. Interestingly that interaction began similarly to the one above, with the physician assuming this was a simple dosage adjustment situation. However, upon hearing the comment, "I get the numbers mixed up," he switched gears to the open-ended question: "So, how are you taking your different insulins?" That inquiry changed the focus of the interview from trying to nail down what the patient had been taking to assessing the extent to which his problems were related to a deficit in skills and abilities. This led to a plan to provide special services, including pre-filled syringes, to address the patient's actual needs.

The fourth axis pertained to habits of deferring care planning until after further testing or consultation with specialists, versus starting to plan care immediately. Physicians who performed well at contextualizing care were generally more likely to make recommendations or decisions about care plans during the visit, whereas those less attentive to context were more inclined to defer decisions to specialists or to discourage patients' questions until they could get their biomedical information needs met. In essence, they were inclined to "kick the can down the road." At the extreme end of the spectrum, a visit would consist of a triage exercise concluding with referrals to several consultants, and orders to get various tests done, with no other substantive discussion. For instance, Dr. B. combined a fast paced "checklisting" approach—"Do you drink? Do you have dark colored stools? . . ."—with rapid fire test ordering. When the patient tried to ask a question about what might be going on, the doctor cut him off with, "I want to do some blood work on you before we talk." She seemed emphatic and impatient with questions, frequently interrupting or finishing the patient's sentences for him. Interestingly, this same clinician also had the computer system mastered, with just brief interludes in interrogations as she paused to enter an order. Hence, it was not as if she had to rush the patient along because of time lost to data entry.

At the same time, Dr. B. indulged in what seemed a bit like voyeurism. As patients revealed their challenges with depression or family hardship, she would want to hear more . . . but sounded more like an inquisitive aunt than a clinician, sometimes passing judgment on what she heard, and not relating it to the patient's care. Our research team members who listened to her audio-recordings wrote that "the doctor seems gossipy." One observed that although "she got very interested in the patient's depression," she did not pick up on clues "even when the USP threw them at the doctor at just the right moment."

In contrast to the, "I want to do some blood work before we talk," orientation of physician Dr. B., Dr. P. attempted to map a plan at each visit, even before test results were in or the diagnosis was clear. Where Dr. B. would take a "let's wait and see what the tests show" approach, Dr. P. would start rendering care right away. For the diabetes patient, for instance, she attended to the confusion and struggles with self-management of a chronic condition by arranging for a diabetes nutrition educator to meet with him that day. During another visit, although she did not initially acknowledge a patient's comment that he was jobless, it clearly registered with her because near the end of the encounter she asked whether he could afford a particular medication. Although Dr. P. is not a "care deferrer," she is also not a "premature closer." She still orders tests, acknowledging that certain things will not be ascertainable until there is more information. But that does not stop her from exploring the relevance of patient context. Such physicians implicitly recognize that, in contrast to biomedical decision-making, which often requires ordering and waiting for test results to take action, contextual information is a continuous stream. They appreciate that each visit is a time to figure out "what is the best next thing for *this* patient at *this* time." Patients struggle with the challenges of managing their care, regardless of whether the diagnosis or the therapeutic plan has been defined.

Although Dr. P. is both attentive to context and mindful of the need for clinical information to inform biomedical decision-making, she does get distracted by the computer. This seems to be something she is aware of, given that she apologetically explains to a couple of patients that she will be typing and looking at the screen during the visit. Her ability to tame the computer-beast, however, varies. For instance, several times she concludes by summarizing something the patient had said while she was typing, but she gets it wrong. On the plus side, her summaries give the patient an opportunity to correct these errors. Regardless, despite the corrections, the typing seemed to disrupt her processing capabilities, because she sometimes failed to incorporate contextual information she had elicited into the care plan. As a result, Dr. P. fell into the middle category among the three groups of physicians in terms of her 4C rated performance at contextualizing care.

Whereas the first four axes have to do with what one might call habits of mind—for example, whether one is rigid or flexible, goes by checklists or follows the narrative, quickly fixes on a diagnosis or remains open-minded, or prefers to wait for all the data before acting or provides care immediately—the fifth axis is more about distractibility and capacity to multitask. Specifically, it has to do with the clinician's ability to manage both the electronic medical record and the patient at the same time. The effort of typing to document the visit while it is occurring is a cognitive drain that draws the clinician's attention away from the patient. For instance, the research team members repeatedly refer to Dr. E.'s typing as a backdrop to all of his encounters. Listening to one visit, a research assistant notes: "Lots of typing, both during breaks and while the patient is talking . . . . The doctor seems hamstrung by the electronic records." They note that the physician appears not to hear what the patient is trying to tell him. In fact, on two occasions the USP actually repeated red flags a couple of times, even though they were not supposed to do this. Presumably, they instinctively reacted to the sense that they were not being heard. Another research assistant notes about the same physician: "Right from the beginning of appointments, there is a lot of typing, with long pauses as the physician seemed to be waiting for the computer screen."

Clinicians who invested so much attention into their interactions with the computer seemed disconnected from patients. For example, the physician might ask a question the patient had already addressed. Sometimes physicians seemed to have stopped listening or even hearing as they focused on whatever data entry task they were trying to accomplish. Instances in which a comment such as "It's been tough since I've lost my job," were followed with a checklist question, such as "Do you have any allergies?" almost always occurred when physicians were distracted by the electronic medical record. Of note, these doctors also tended to be systems reviewers rather than theory builders, perhaps because overattention to the computer and working one's way through checklists go hand-in-hand.

On the other end of the spectrum were doctors who interacted as if there were no computer in the room. Without a video recording, we can only speculate as to how these clinicians functioned so well. One approach some doctors adopt is to prepare in advance of visits, by looking over the medical records of scheduled patients at the start of the day, and formatting notes in advance. This is accomplished by cutting and pasting information from previous notes that is not likely to have changed. The Veterans Health Administration (VA) electronic medical records system, the Computerized Patient Records System (CPRS), also has features that, with a few clicks of the mouse, enable providers to import the latest medication list, vitals, and previously documented medical problems into the note template. Hence, those physicians who have the time and inclination can free themselves of some of the distraction of doing this work during an encounter.

Unshackled from the computer, clinicians were more likely to relax and engage. Listening to physician Dr. G., one hears some typing, but otherwise one would not know he is working on a computer. The clinician is quite structured, even beginning with a checklist, but the visit seems more relaxed. Although he is checklist oriented, there is room for conversation. In addition, the clinician seems to be processing what he is hearing, noting for instance what he and the patient have already discussed about eating habits when he gets to the diet section of his interview with a veteran who has diabetes.

Despite being a good listener, and not overwhelmed by data entry, Dr. G. is strikingly lacking in conventional social courtesy. He does not introduce himself at the start of the visit or greet the patient. But he does pick up on transportation issues and challenges for the patient of getting to a specialist, and received a high score for contextualized care planning. Attending to the patient rather than the computer, while essential to care planning, does not ensure good "bedside manner."

Although the ability to keep the voracious demands of the computer at bay and the patient at the fore of the visit is a critical trait, and one that is associated with high performance at contextualizing care, it does not necessarily signify an affinity for building relationships with patients. Clinicians such as Dr. G. illustrate how certain traits that we tend to think will go together, such as good communication behavior and effective care delivery, do not entirely overlap. On the one hand, we have observed doctors who lack social graces but are laser-like in their focus on what the patient says and needs. On the other, are the schmoozers who love to talk but nonetheless miss the clues or overt concerns of patients.

When we explored how physicians who contextualize care differ from those who do not, we sought to identify a set of characteristics that were all inclusive, so that every physician would fit at least one of them. That led to the five axes. But then we listened to encounters with a physician such as Dr. C., who is far above average at contextualizing care but in other respects is pretty unlikeable. His visits with patients are humorless and directive. He controls the visit, avoiding small talk and asking strings of questions interrupted by long pauses as he enters data into the medical record. Our team could not classify him as flexible, nor could they say that he is a theory builder. Although he is not prone to premature closure, he also is not particularly open-minded. It is true that he avoids deferring care, but this is primarily a consequence of successfully identifying contextual issues that compel action. Hence, we created a sixth and final axis, which acknowledges the fact that some people just recognize the import of context more than others for reasons we do not yet understand. This six and final axis, then, extends from the noncontextual to the contextual thinker. Noncontextual thinkers simply do not connect the dots linking a contextual red flag to the patient's presenting problem. For instance, in the case of the patient who came to the doctor with a complaint about his worsening asthma, even while taking an expensive brand name medication, and commented that things had been tough since he lost his job, some docs just did not make a connection, despite a discussion about the contextual issue. In one case, the physician engaged the patient in a rambling conversation about how difficult the job market had become, with the patient commenting that he did not have any immediate job prospects, and the physician still did not ask about any trouble paying for Pulmicort, which costs $185 a month. Without an appreciation for the relevance of context to planning care, none of the other axes matter. Interestingly, this same physician thought about the stress associated with being unemployed and commented that stress might be exacerbating the asthma through its biomedical effects on smooth muscle relaxation in the chest. But the possibility that the word "tough" in the patient's comment might mean something specific about the patient's life challenge, and its impact on his ability to care for himself, did not seem to occur to this doctor.

The best contextual thinkers, in contrast, not only explore the implications of life challenges for care planning when they hear the red flag, but then also assimilate them into all of their planning for the rest of the visit. One physician, Dr. H., after asking about the patient's ability to pay for his medication upon hearing that things have been tough since he lost his job, also considered the implications of lack of insurance later in the encounter as he weighed whether or not to send the patient for pulmonary function testing:

> DOCTOR: "... One thing I was a little bit worried, for your sake, is you know, doctors ... we order a lot of tests ...."
> PATIENT: "Yeah."
> DOCTOR: "And I don't want to get you in a situation where you're having to, you know, choose between, uh, doing whatever it is that I come up with or I recommend and paying for it."
> PATIENT: "Got you."

The physician's awkwardness is palpable as he broaches a subject that makes him uncomfortable, but one senses that he mainly is concerned about not embarrassing the patient, as well as respecting the patient's financial challenges as they plan care. At the most basic level, however, he recognizes and can generalize the implications of context in care planning.

Taken together, these axes illustrate the cognitive behaviors that differentiate physicians who effectively address context in care planning from those who do not, and reveal that most fall somewhere along a continuum across six sets of characteristics. The archetype of a clinician who exemplifies all of the skills for attending to the complexity of context in decision-making is an individual who is flexible rather than rigid in conversation, does not let checklists get in the way of building and testing theories about what might be going on, avoids drawing conclusions prematurely in the face of conflicting evidence, looks for opportunities in every visit to provide some level of care to the patient right now, manages rather than is managed by technology, and is capable of seeing the link- ages between patients' life situations and their clinical care. Conversely, the archetype of the physician who overlooks context is an individual who must drive the interview according to his or her assumptions about what is important, is not easily diverted from a set of routinized questions, reaches conclusions about what is going on and what needs to be done based on the information obtained from a narrow biomedical perspec- tive, regards care planning as a last step rather than an ongoing process in patient care, is distracted and controlled by data entry, and sees patient context as a curiosity, distraction, or chance to build rapport rather than as data relevant to care planning. Using the same 1 to 10 scale employed in our analysis, Figure 5.2 shows that the highest performing physicians are closest to the first archetype across five of the six axes (darkest line), the lowest are closest to the second archetype (light grey) and the middle performers (medium grey) fall between these two groups, overlapping with the lowest performers on electronic medical record skill.

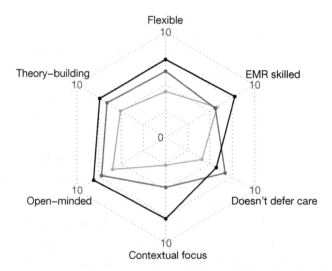

Figure 5.2
Comparing low (light grey line), middle (medium grey line), and high (black line) performers on six dimensions.

What would it take to move clinicians closer to the former archetype and away from the latter? Are these skills teachable? Are all clinicians capable of learning, or only those who already exhibit a capacity to think contextually? Where can one intervene in the professional development of the clinician to address the problem? Should it be in practice, residency training, or medical school, or during the admissions process? Can changes to the way we use technology make a difference? How much of the solution requires training or retraining how doctors think versus changing how quality-of-care is defined and measured? Finally, how might one begin to tackle these questions?

We began our examination of these questions with a narrowly constructed but rigorous study. We asked whether simply teaching clinicians—at an early formative stage in their careers—about the importance of contextualizing care, providing them with an opportunity to see how it makes a difference for the care of their own patients, and giving them a chance to practice a new set of skills, would make a measurable difference. We studied this educational intervention as if we were studying a pill in a clinical trial. In the next chapter we describe this experiment.

Better Teaching, Better Doctors

"I'm so glad I asked . . . ."
—*Medical student in workshop on contextualizing care after hearing that
her patient would have declined a lifesaving heart valve repair because
"there is no one to hold my hand and support me after the surgery."*

We had learned that contextualizing care requires more than longer visits or empathic communication styles. In reviewing the transcripts of practicing physicians faced with our actors, we realized that contextualizing care was a set of communication and thinking skills. The physician needs to know the right kinds of questions to ask, needs to ask those questions, needs to listen carefully to the patient's answers, needs to understand what these answers reveal about their patient's life circumstances, needs to think about how those circumstances affect the patient, and needs to think about how care should be arranged to accommodate these circumstances.

If these are really communication and thinking skills, they are not being acquired by physicians during their training. Both of us are deeply involved in medical education, so naturally, we next asked why physicians had not learned these skills, and whether we could teach medical students and residents to be better at contextualizing care.

THE MAKING OF A DOCTOR

The training of physicians in the United States is long and complex. Consider what goes into the making of a general internist, the most common kind of physician seeing adult patients (especially those with chronic diseases) for both regular checkups and illnesses.

The usual course of premedical training is a four-year college degree, often with a major in a biological or behavioral science that provides some grounding in the scientific processes of life, as well as the scientific method of research. In chemistry, for example, the student learns that the way chemical elements react follows an elegant and consistent set of rules. In biology, the student comes to see the common processes that underlie basic functions like respiration and metabolism. In psychology, the student is taught that behavior can be understood and explained through properly designed experiments and the application of statistical methods to separate real causes and effects from coincidences and random associations.

Admission to medical school most often is based on a combination of grades, test scores, personal essays, letters of recommendation, and interviews. The most important of these is usually the Medical College Admission Test (MCAT), a standardized test consisting largely of multiple choice questions focused on biological and physical science knowledge (and, more recently, a smattering of social science). Of the others, only the interview purports to measure the prospective medical student's ability to interact with others. Unfortunately, in the traditional medical school admission interview, the applicants answer the questions rather than ask them. A growing trend, originating in Canada, seeks to replace the traditional interview with the Multiple Mini Interview (MMI) consisting of about nine stations through which candidates cycle briefly. At each station they are challenged to respond to scenarios that assess what are termed "soft skills," such as professionalism, interpersonal communication, ethical behavior, empathy, and emotional intelligence. Interestingly, candidates are still generally asked to respond to questions rather than formulate them.

What happens once the applicant becomes a medical student? For decades, U.S. medical schools have divided their four-year curricula into roughly two parts. Two "preclinical years," focused on basic sciences such as anatomy, pathology, and physiology, are followed by two "clinical years," in which students work with doctors in clinics, hospitals, and other healthcare settings to help take care of patients. The clinical years usually are organized into required and elective clerkships by specialties—12 weeks of internal medicine, 8 weeks of pediatrics, 6 weeks of obstetrics/gynecology, 12 weeks of surgery, etc. To progress from the preclinical to clinical years requires passing the United States Medical Licensing Exam (USMLE) Step 1 test, another standardized test focused on basic science knowledge.

One thing that medical schools have discovered is that when the two preclinical years focus exclusively on learning and testing basic science facts, students set aside their laudable aspirations as healers in favor of mastering the biological mechanisms of health and illness. In response, most schools now introduce limited interactions with patients, such as interviewing a patient and taking a medical history, during the preclinical years, often as part of an ongoing course called "essentials of clinical medicine," "introduction to clinical medicine," "art of medicine," or "doctoring."

At the end of the clinical years, our would-be internist takes another exam, the USMLE Step 2, which contains a clinical knowledge portion and a clinical skills portion. The clinical knowledge portion is another fact-based multiple choice exam. The clinical skills portion includes encounters with several standardized patients, and is used to assess communication skills and clinical judgment.

Graduation from a medical school with an MD or DO degree grants one the title of "doctor." The degree alone, however, is not enough to be licensed as a practicing physician in the United States. Our young doctor must now specialize by completing a residency program. As a resident, she or he will, under the supervision of a practicing attending physician, be directly responsible for the care of patients in and out of the hospital. A residency in internal medicine consists of three core years of training, after which the graduate is eligible to be licensed by a state medical board for private practice as a general internist and to take the American Board of Internal Medicine's certifying examination (another multiple-choice test) to be recognized as a "board-certified" internist. Physicians who want to subspecialize (e.g., in cardiology), must engage in additional subspecialty fellowship training, which requires not only patient care but research training.

Where in this training is contextualization of care formally taught? Nowhere. The lucky patient has a physician whose clerkship preceptors and residency supervisors emphasized and modeled attention to patients' individual circumstances. But as we saw in our USP studies, few supervising physicians have these skills themselves.

In short, most medical education places heavy emphasis on scientific evidence and biomedical decision-making with little emphasis on how to incorporate contextual factors that are essential to planning patient care. Trainees learn to consider rare diseases or unusual presentations of more common diseases, but are offered no comparable framework for considering the boundless complexity of a patient's life. The same can be said for the assessment of clinical performance. Trainees typically are tested at diagnosing the signs and symptoms of disease, and on pairing that diagnosis with recommended management. There is, however, no systematic approach to gauging trainees' skills at tailoring care to patients' needs and circumstances.

HOW TO TEACH CONTEXTUALIZATION OF CARE

When we began to think about teaching contextualization, we realized that biomedical and contextual reasoning skills are distinct. Biomedical reasoning—what medical students spend nearly all of their time learning—involves categorization, or figuring out the "box" into which to fit a patient. Does this patient have diabetes? What type? What medications can be used? Contextual reasoning, on the other hand, requires discovery—understanding how a patient is unique.[1],2 Why does this patient have trouble controlling her sugars? What kinds of medications actually are available to her? And which are possible for her to use, given her daily routines?

We wanted our students to hear their patients and develop meaningful interpretations of their life context and its relationship with their health care. In many ways, the discovery process we outlined for contextualizing care is similar to an approach to research often referred to as "qualitative."[3] Unlike quantitative methods, which seek to measure causes and effects and describe their relationships mathematically, qualitative methods seek to discover the meaning of observations in their rich original, often textual or narrative, state without reducing them to numbers. In designing and teaching a curriculum on contextualization of care, we worked with Ilene Harris, Professor and Head of the University of Illinois at Chicago (UIC) Department of Medical Education, and an expert both in medical education and qualitative research methods.

Because contextual thinking cuts across clinical specialties and is not limited to any particular basic science course (it does not fit cleanly into the existing educational "boxes"), we looked for an opportunity for students to focus on context and contextual reasoning. But the medical school curriculum is a busy one, and there is little room for adding new courses. To demonstrate that learning about contextualization of care could improve student skills, we had to make the most of very limited teaching time. We also had to find the right place in the curriculum to insert the material. Our aim was to design a brief hands-on curriculum to help medical students develop knowledge and skills in contextualizing patient care at a time when they would be most receptive and available.[1],3

We concluded that the best place would be near the end of medical school, in the fourth year, both because that is where there is more flexibility in the curriculum and also because it would come at a time when students no longer are preoccupied with learning the basics of how to examine a medical patient, make a diagnosis, and formulate a treatment plan. We also wanted to do the teaching in a setting where students could apply what they learned in real time to real patients. Hence, we organized a set of four weekly one-hour sessions to occur during the required fourth-year "subinternship" in internal medicine. Subinterns function almost like interns (first-year residents) in that they admit and manage their own patients in the hospital, but with more supervision than a full-fledged intern.

In the first two sessions of the minicurriculum on contextualizing care, students learned about concepts and terms through discussions of cases, and in the second two sessions they applied what they learned to their actual patients. We began with an overview of medical decision-making; few medical students, or fully fledged physicians for that matter, have had an opportunity in their formal education to think about the process explicitly. (We find it surprising that the one thing that nearly all physicians do all the time—make medical decisions—is not taught. Given that one of us is editor of the journal, *Medical Decision Making*, this is, perhaps, a sore point). In the 1990s, a team based mainly at McMaster University in Canada, which had pioneered the evidence-based medicine (EBM) movement discussed in Chapter 2, characterized good medical decision-making, which they termed "clinical expertise," as the integration of three distinct types of information. First, one needs to know about a patient's "clinical state," which refers to everything going on that is biomedical, that is, everything going on inside the body. This knowledge comes from looking over the medical record, taking a good medical history, conducting a physical exam, and ordering lab tests and other studies. The description of a patient's clinical state might include that she has diabetes and hypertension, that her diabetes is quite well controlled, but her blood pressure remains high despite her use of an antihypertensive medication.

The second type of information involved in clinical expertise is the "research evidence," which refers to the best science available that is pertinent to the patient's clinical state. What do clinical trials tell us, for instance, about how best to manage someone who has high blood pressure that is not responsive to single drug therapy, and who also happens to have diabetes? There are actually a lot of studies on this specific question. Once one has identified the research evidence to manage a particular clinical state, in essence one has a diagnosis and treatment. At this point, it is easy to think, especially if one is a busy clinician, that one has done one's homework and it is time to move on. Yet, at least one—and we argue two—additional pieces of information are still needed.

The third type of information in the EBM model is the patient's preferences. Nearly all treatments have potential side effects and risks, and information about whether those risks outweigh the potential benefits only can come from the person who will be subjected to those risks and benefits. Let us now give our hypothetical patient with hypertension and diabetes a name, as she ceases to be just a disease once we introduce individual preferences. We will call her Ms. Sanders. For the physician who is trying to get Ms. Sanders's blood pressure down a few notches into the normal range, choosing another medication from among a list of available options is just a moment's thought. Often the decision is made based on the doctor's comfort level with several of the options that he or she has prescribed for years. For Ms. Sanders, however, the decision is about a little pill she will take at least daily; a pill that will send new chemicals to nearly every cell in her body continuously for perhaps the rest of her life. If her blood pressure is just above goal, she may prefer to forgo additional medication and attempt nonpharmacological strategies through dietary changes and exercise. But she may only consider that option if it is offered to her. Doctors are taught that they should pay attention to patient wishes, but few are trained to recognize that eliciting patient preferences is a systematic part of clinical decision-making.

Our work introduces a fourth type of information to the decision-making—patient context. One might argue that if physicians allow patients to exercise their preferences, they will instinctively take into account the contextual factors in their lives that are relevant to their care. For instance, if Ms. Sanders has inadequate healthcare coverage, she is likely to prefer a less expensive antihypertensive medicine over a more expensive one, if given the choice. However, if she is a long-haul truck driver, she may not be aware that certain blood pressure medications induce more frequent urination, particularly during the first few weeks as one's body adapts to them, and could cause significant discomfort on the road. She would have to rely on the physician to figure out what information is relevant about her life situation, or context, to making an optimal medical decision.

Introducing patient context to students by showing how it is part of a larger thinking process allowed us to establish a conceptual foundation for understanding its place in the clinical encounter. "Patient context" is not just one more thing to worry about when one is caring for patients, it is the missing fourth leg of a table—the surface upon which we arrive at a plan of care (Figure 6.1).

When one of us first made this argument in a 2004 paper, Brian Haynes, a McMaster scholar who pioneered EBM, generously invited an editorial in "ACP Journal Club" arguing for the role of context in decision-making. ACP Journal Club summarizes the best new clinically relevant research and disseminates it to every member of the American College of Physicians with occasional accompanying conceptual pieces. Titled "From research evidence to context: the challenge of individualizing care," the article walks the reader through a case example of an elderly

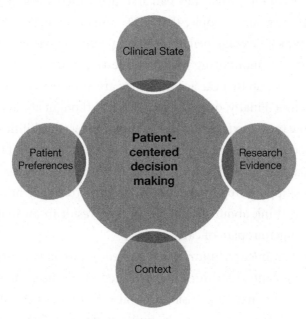

Figure 6.1
Adding context to models of clinical expertise.

gentleman whose clinical state includes a diagnosis of atrial fibrillation for which the research evidence shows a benefit of providing the antico-agulant warfarin, because it can slightly reduce the chances of having a stroke. Although the patient would prefer not to have a stroke, putting him on warfarin also increases the chances that he will have a serious bleed if he falls down. The chances of a serious fall seem to be substantial, given that he lives alone in a home where he has slipped on stairs twice. In addition, he already is taking another medication that can augment the bleeding risk of warfarin. Should this man take warfarin?

We began the first of the four sessions with one of several similar cases that illustrate how arriving at an appropriate care plan requires consideration of context. It is particularly effective to begin by presenting only information about the clinical state and asking the students what they would do. Most of them have diligently learned the relevant research evidence so they are eager to respond. Then, we would throw in a twist by asking them about patient preferences and revealing what the patient actually said he wanted. Our students would discover that patients do not necessarily prefer what they had assumed patients would prefer. Not everyone thinks, for example, that a 2% annual reduction in risk of a stroke—a typical average benefit of taking warfarin—is worth the hassle of continuous monitoring with blood testing and the risk that if they fall down or end up in a car accident they are at increased probability of severe bleeding. Finally, once the students had thought about all that, we would throw in contextual factors—competing responsibilities, financial challenges, the loss of social support, etc.—and ask them what they would do. Our goal was to walk novice clinicians through a process that illustrates how skipping steps, particularly the ones that they have not been sensitized to think about systematically, can result in an inappropriate and even dangerous plan of care.

Hence, our minicurriculum was designed to provide a foundation for incorporating contextual thinking into medical decision-making. Over the course of the first two sessions, we also introduced the 10 domains of patient context and provided examples to illustrate how each domain could alter what makes sense in the care of a particular patient. We drew analogies from traditional biomedical decision-making concepts. For instance, medical students routinely are taught to formulate a *differential diagnosis* for their patients—a list of possible causes of a patient's symptoms in order of likelihood—and to use their differential diagnosis to guide their reasoning process. The differential diagnosis for worsening asthma includes new allergic triggers, gastroesophageal reflux disease, and viral infections. We taught them to develop a *contextual differential* as well, in which they were to consider, in order of likelihood, the possible domains of context that could contribute to their patient's problems. They were to use those possible domains to guide their contextual reasoning and help them identify which domains might actually be involved. The contextual differential for worsening asthma includes financial factors impacting on ability to purchase medications, competing responsibilities interfering with medical administration, and knowledge and skills deficits regarding how to take medication correctly. Finally, we integrated these concepts and terms into a series of steps that would later become our coding system, "Content Coding for Contextualization of Care" (4C). Our students learned to be on the lookout for contextual *red flags*, to probe for contextual factors, and to incorporate what they learned into the care plan.

The second two sessions took students, and what they had learned, literally to the bedside. We began in the conference rooms, located on the medicine wards, where they were accustomed to meeting. Instead of pulling out another case, we would ask them to talk about patients they had admitted during the prior 24 hours. For each, we would challenge them to identify a contextual red flag. Some of the stories told in earlier chapters came from these sessions. For instance, the opening account in Chapter 1 of Amelia Garcia originated from a student presentation and follow-up bedside visit. Ms. Garcia had been admitted the previous night for hemodialysis with her usual fluid overload and electrolyte abnormalities. She would have gone home that afternoon with no follow-up plan other than the usual admonishment not to miss her hemodialysis again in the future. However, a student participating in our educational intervention recognized, following a discussion of the case, that this patient's recurring ER visits for a preventable problem was a contextual red flag. With some new conceptual tools in hand, she made her way with our team in tow to the patient's room, where she interviewed Ms. Garcia with help from a bilingual classmate.

The educational value of these bedside learning experiences—apart from their obvious quality-of-care benefit for patients—is that they were an epiphany for students. The students had seen the patient admitted and analyzed and assessed by multiple physicians and other staff to arrive at what seemed to be an appropriate care plan. And then to discover that major issues had been overlooked and that the care plan was actually inappropriate—that turned on a light bulb. The extent to which these "Aha" moments appeared to have the desired effect varied considerably from student to student. "M4s," as they are called, are already well along in being indoctrinated into a particular narrow biomedical model. While for one student, the discovery that Ms. Garcia had been repeatedly admitted and put at risk unnecessarily because nobody thought to find out that she needed to have her dialysis moved to a more convenient location was a big deal, for another student it just was not of interest. In fact, some students were offended and found it inappropriate that we were returning to patients' bedsides to ask them questions when we were not a part of the care team, even when the attending in charge of the patient and the patient had given consent. It was as if all the attention to the patients' psychosocial situations, and the intimate questions this entailed, seemed somehow off to them. Reactions sometimes bordered on hostile.

We did ask students why they thought they and their teams tended not to explore patient context, and we got essentially four answers. The first was that they do not like asking questions when they think they will not know what to do with the answers. The second is that once we ask patients about their life situations, it opens a Pandora's box, and there are too many other things to deal with already. The third answer we received is that asking patients about their life situations could trigger a lot of emotion to pour out, and the students feared they would not be comfortable with that. And fourth, some said that they just did not think it was their job.

Medical training reinforces the notion that learning and practicing medicine is about applying knowledge from fields such as biochemistry, physiology, and pathology to prescribe treatments or preventions for various conditions. There is also a variable amount of teaching about communication behavior, medical ethics, and professionalism, but these concepts do not seem to translate into an understanding of the broader goals of caring for patients. Our hope was that this brief educational intervention would serve as a jolt against the prevailing current. We were interested to see whether it was having any effect.

TESTING THE TEACHING

Teaching contextualization successfully would mean that the students become skilled at probing contextual red flags and incorporating contextual factors in care planning. We wanted to show convincingly that these were learnable skills and that even our brief workshop could improve them measurably.

A simple approach would be to teach some students these skills and then test them using standardized patients. At UIC, as at most medical schools, and as part of USMLE Step 2, our students were already being assessed for a variety of skills with standardized patients, so they were accustomed to the idea. In fact, because we still were working with the actors from our USP study, we could ask the same actors to portray the same cases that we had used in the USP study—cases we already knew posed challenges for practicing physicians. We could give some students the workshop, and subsequently have them perform visits with the standardized patients in our clinical performance center, and see whether they successfully contextualized care.

"But wait," a successful student might say, "How would you know that your workshop is how I learned to do that? Maybe I was already good at contextualizing care?" One way we could address this objection would be to test the student before and after the workshop. "But wait," an actor might say, "If I present the same case twice to the same student, won't they recognize the case and improve the second time?"

In clinical research, the strongest form of evidence for the value of a new practice is to conduct a randomized controlled trial. Take a group of patients who might benefit from the new practice, divide them randomly into two groups, and give only one group the new practice. Give the other group the standard practice (which may be no treatment at all), or something that resembles the new practice superficially but does not contain some key features (e.g., administering a lookalike placebo instead of a drug). Measure the outcomes for each group, and if the new practice group does better than the other group, we have a strong argument that it is the new practice itself that is responsible for better outcomes, rather than pre-existing differences (which would be equalized between the groups by dividing them randomly) or simply improvement over time (which would be similar in both groups).

The same standards can be applied to educational research. Take a group of students from the same medical school and provide a contextualization workshop to half of them, chosen at random. Test both groups with standardized patients, and see whether the workshop group outperforms the other group.

Designing and conducting a randomized trial is not easy or cheap, and one reason there are so many fewer educational than clinical trials is that there are fewer sources of funding for educational research. However, the National Board of Medical Examiners—the developers of the USMLE tests—has a Center for Innovation that annually awards one to two Edward J. Stemmler, MD Medical Education Research Fund grants. These grants reflect NBME's sustained commitment to studying and improving methods for assessing medical skills. We were fortunate to obtain a Stemmler Grant, which enabled us to conduct our study using the fourth-year medical student class at UIC.

For 15 months, during month-long internal medicine subinternships at two neighboring hospitals, we taught the contextualization workshop at one hospital and not at the other. We alternated hospitals for the workshop to separate the effect of the workshop from the effect of the clinical site. Medical students at UIC are assigned to their subinternship months and hospitals based on a random lottery process, with six to eight students per hospital per month. By repeating the workshop with half the students each month, we made sure that both groups had students earlier and later in their medical training.

At the end of each month, both groups of students came to our clinical performance center and interviewed four standardized patients—the same four cases and actors that we had used in the USP study described earlier. And as in the USP study, we measured whether students noticed and probed both biomedical and contextual red flags, and whether they incorporated unusual biomedical and contextual factors, when present, into their care plans. We took special care to be sure that the people who were listening to recordings of the interviews or reviewing the students' care plans had no knowledge of whether the student had been in a workshop group or not.

We hoped (and expected) that students who had been in the workshop would be better than those who had not been at probing contextual red flags and at contextualizing their care plans when they discovered a contextual factor. We hoped we would not see any difference in probing biomedical red flags or incorporating biomedical factors into care plans, because we did not want to make students worse at biomedical reasoning as a result of less focus and practice on biomedical reasoning during our workshop.

Our results were heartening. We had 124 students participate in the study and the standardized patient assessments. Students who had taken the workshop probed contextual red flags 86% of the time, while those who had not only probed them 61% of the time. For biomedical red flags, however, both groups probed them 77% of the time. Similarly, students who had taken the workshop contextualized their care plans in 67% of the encounters with a contextual factor, while those who had not taken the workshop only contextualized in 24% of these encounters. Again, there was no difference among the two groups in adapting care plans to biomedical factors. Further analysis showed that although probing for context made contextual planning more likely, the workshop group was better at planning than the other students, even in cases in which both groups probed. We published these results in *JAMA: The Journal of the American Medical Association*, and the journal featured our study in its *JAMA Report* video series.[4]

We were happy to find that medical students could demonstrate improvement after even a brief introduction to contextualization of care. We introduced the same workshop and conducted a second randomized trial with resident physicians and standardized patients as part of our study audio-recording real patient encounters described in Chapter 3. Once again, as measured with standardized patients, residents who had received our four-hour workshop were more likely to contextualize their care plan (65% for workshop participants vs. 43% for others).

THE GAP BETWEEN COMPETENCE AND PERFORMANCE

We had proven that we could teach medical students and residents enough about contextualization that they could demonstrate improved skills when tested. That is, we had improved the competence of our learners. Competence is necessary for successful performance—if one does not know how to do something correctly, one will not reliably do it correctly. But competence is not the same as performance. We can know how to draw a bow and hit a target alone at an indoor archery range, but doing the same in an outdoor archery competition in the face of wind and other competitors may be substantially more difficult.

Our workshop study with the medical students led to an ironic discovery in this vein. We had used the same cases and actors to test our students as we had in the USP study with practicing physicians. Table 6.1 compares the success of our trained students, our untrained students, and the practicing physicians.

Not only did our trained students do better at contextual probing and care planning than the practicing physicians, our untrained students were better as well. But that is not because medical students are better than attending physicians—it is because the medical students who succeed

TABLE 6.1 COMPARISON OF PROBING AND PLANNING RATES AMONG
STUDENTS (WITH STANDARDIZED PATIENTS) AND PRACTICING
PHYSICIANS (WITH UNANNOUNCED STANDARDIZED PATIENTS)

	Trained Students/ Tested in Lab	Untrained Students/ Tested in Lab	Practicing Physicians/ USPs in their offices
Biomedical Probing	77%	77%	65%
Contextual Probing	86%	60%	46%
Correct Care Plan	61%	50%	33%

are demonstrating competence in a controlled situation when they know
they are being tested, while the practicing physicians who succeed are
demonstrating real-world performance when they do not know they are
being tested. That is a higher standard and a harder test.

In 1990, George Miller, one of the founding figures in the study of medical education, proposed a four-level hierarchy of assessment, popularly
called "Miller's Pyramid." The hierarchy is "knows," "knows how," "shows
how," and "does." Each succeeding level is more important and more difficult to assess. We had proven our workshop improved contextualization
at the "shows how" level; learners could demonstrate contextual care with
standardized patients. But we also knew that seeing an effect on performance outside of testing conditions—the "does" level—would be much
more valuable. In our study with residents and real patients, we had the
opportunity to look at the "does" level, because, as described in Chapter 3,
we had measured their contextualization skills and their real patients'
outcomes over the following nine months. We knew that contextualized
care resulted in better patient outcomes, but did the residents who had
our workshop contextualize care more often with their real patients?

Unfortunately, no. In the audiotapes where our team heard contextual
red flags, residents probed those flags 27% of the time, whether or not
they had been through our workshop. When our team heard contextual factors that should have been incorporated into care plans, residents

incorporated those factors 34% of the time, whether or not they had taken the workshop. And, as a result, the health outcomes of the patients, which we knew got better when their doctors contextualized care plans, were no different in the two groups.

Thus one of the lessons of this chapter is that although we can improve skills with a minicourse, without a more powerful approach, we cannot in four hours of training transform how physicians approach their daily work. Real change requires frequent assessment with feedback, based on what is observed in actual practice. Furthermore, altering something as complex as how doctors take care of patients requires frequent reinforcement. We concluded that to make all this happen we would need to continue to enlist actual patients to audio-record their encounters, and to provide ongoing and meaningful feedback to the doctors themselves.

Is Lasting Change Possible?

"Wow, my grandmother could do better than this. She has common sense."
—Comment by an attending physician after reviewing a report based on
audio-recordings of physician interactions with patients in her clinic.

When callers reach any number of companies for customer service or tech support, they hear a recording saying, "This call may be recorded for quality assurance." The process is referred to as "audit and feedback." Employees are told, essentially, "When you work here you will occasionally be recorded while assisting our customers." The purpose is to assess their performance-in-practice, rather than just review what they have been taught to do. There are scoring systems for evaluating how employees perform based on the audios collected. Those scoring systems can influence what we hear as customers when we make those phone calls. When an Internet cable service agent repeatedly asks us at the end of a call if he has fully addressed all of our needs and whether there is anything else he can possibly do to help us, it is clear that someone has given him a script to follow. Although exasperating at times, the process does have its advantages. Contrast this experience with, for instance, exchanges with a front-line bureaucrat at a post office, airline baggage claim, or emergency department when nobody else is listening.

Most of us have experienced rudeness or indifference as a response to our requests for assistance, and wished for some accountability.

Such audio-based audit and feedback, however, generally has been reserved for customer service workers providing phone support rather than for professionals in practice. Professionals are not supposed to need this kind of scrutiny because, after all, they are professionals. The argument against audit and feedback, presumably, is that it is not necessary—that because of their extensive training, and acculturation to their vocation, professionals are self-regulating and hold themselves to the highest standard, obviating the need for such oversight. After analyzing thousands of encounters between physicians and patients, we are not convinced.

Professionals delivering health services are, in fact, evaluated. Uncommon two decades ago, nearly all physicians now are tracked with an ever-growing set of metrics. Broadly speaking, these metrics fall into two categories: process measures and outcome measures. Process measures include tracking of the order of tests or treatments that are considered appropriate for a particular clinical situation based on research evidence. For instance, many studies show that a category of blood pressure medicine called beta blockers can reduce mortality if given to people who have had heart attacks. So, it is relatively straightforward to see whether patients who have a diagnosis of myocardial infarction noted in their chart subsequently have been put on beta blockers. Another example of a process measure is seeing whether screening tests are delivered to the right individuals at the right times in their lives. This would include colonoscopy and mammography, for instance. These are all process measures because they ascertain whether processes that are known to be efficacious in particular situations are followed.

Outcome measures are more compelling but harder to assess. For instance, documenting not only that a physician's patients who have had heart attacks are getting beta blockers, but that they are living longer than average would be terrific but unrealistic. It would take too many years, and there would be insufficient numbers of patients in a single practice to detect statistically significant differences from norms. Some outcome measures can be, and are, tracked quite often, such as glucose control in patients with diabetes. Physicians often are held accountable not only for getting these patients the right care but for actually getting their disease state under good control.

Physicians have many objections to performance measures, and one of the most compelling is that they tend to reinforce "cookie-cutter" medicine. When a patient walks into a doctor's office, little does he or she know that the doctor probably already has a long agenda in mind. Depending on patient age, medical conditions, and lifestyle issues, there may be quite a list of things that the doctor needs to do to hit her performance goals. On the one hand, this is probably not a good situation for either the doctor or the patient. On the other hand, there is a certain logic to it. Countless clinical trials costing taxpayer money have generated a foundation of evidence to show that various tests and therapies can help people live longer and better if delivered correctly. It is also known that lots of people do not benefit from all the science because their healthcare team neglects to offer them effective care. In particular, there seem to be major disparities according to race and ethnicity in who gets offered beneficial services. This is another reason to track who is getting what care.

Performance measures are probably here to stay, but they can have unintended consequences. For instance, they may promote treating patients as though they were interchangeable. There are relatively recent efforts, however, to customize measures rather than assert a one-size-fits-all approach. For some performance measures, physicians and patients can agree on what they will prioritize and focus on, and the physician is then tracked for success at achieving those shared goals.

What all of these measures have in common is that they are drawn from data that are extracted from the medical record. As far as we are aware, there are not any performance measures that assess the actual real-life, real-time delivery of care. That would require employing some kind of direct observation, such as the methods that we have used in our research: the unannounced standardized patient or real patients who audio-record their visits. As detailed in the previous chapters, the things one learns by directly observing care (or, literally, listening to care) could

not possibly come from chart review. A physician who overlooks a contextual red flag is not going to document what she missed, of course,
because she does not realize what she missed.

But there is another reason that assessing performance based on
directly observed care could be transformative: It is the antidote to
the cookie-cutter problem. Whereas the medical record is the place to
find out what a patient requires that is similar to other patients, the
audio-recorded encounter is where one learns about specific needs.
Because our coding system, "Content Coding for Contextualization of
Care" (4C), is a performance measure of individualization of care, it can
not rely on data from the medical record. Analysis of audio-recorded
data is the only way to know whether clinicians are collecting data
about individual patient circumstances and, in some cases, prudently
discounting guidelines based on those circumstances. For instance, for
patients with multiple chronic illnesses, adhering to all recommended
guidelines for each condition they have could overwhelm them.
Attention to the clues, or contextual red flags, that a patient is unable
to cope with the complexity of his care either because of competing
responsibilities, a lack of skills and abilities, or other contextual factors
will prompt the sensitive and judicious physician to appropriately customize or contextualize care. If traditional performance measures that
promote cookie-cutter care assess what automatons can do, data collected from directly observed care can assess the judgment that intelligent thoughtful professionals exercise.

FROM MEASURING PERFORMANCE TO IMPROVING IT

Of course, it is not helpful to measure performance unless one does
something with the information. The purpose of performance measurement is to drive performance improvement. How does one do this? As
we discussed in the previous chapter, acquiring a skill does not necessarily translate into better practice. It is not enough to teach medical students and physicians to give beta blockers to patients who have had heart

attacks, or to recommend colon cancer screening to patients based on a set of guidelines, and assume that they will then consistently do so. There are well-documented gaps between what doctors are taught and the services patients receive in virtually every area of medical practice where this problem has been studied.

The Veterans Health Administration (VA) has shown that they can close these gaps, or at least narrow them, with continuous performance measurement and feedback. Often that feedback comes with money attached or withheld based on what are termed "performance pay goals." Goals are determined locally within specific clinics at VA facilities based on the health status of the veteran population in the practice. For instance at Jesse Brown VA Medical Center in Chicago, 25% of physician performance pay in 2015 was linked to reductions in the number of veterans with poorly controlled diabetes in each physician's practice. To get all the additional pay, physicians had to drive down the proportion of their patients with a hemoglobin A1c > 9 by at least 20%, or document that less than 20% of their patients with diabetes have not already reached this target.

Performance measurement driven quality improvement seems to work. As early as 2004, a major study comparing veterans' care to care of patients in commercial health insurance plans across 26 medical conditions and 348 quality improvement measures demonstrated both that veterans were getting higher quality care on average and, most significantly, that the difference was greatest in those areas where the VA measures performance.[1]

It should be noted that paying for performance is just one of a number of strategies for using performance data to improve quality. For instance the VA widely uses what are called "clinical reminders." Every time a patient is seen in primary care the cover page of his or her electronic health record shows the various preventive care screening or monitoring tests that are due based on the patient's particular medical and demographic profile. Just letting physicians know with a clinical reminder that it is time to recommend a colonoscopy (or an alternative screening test such as a flexible sigmoidoscopy) may prompt them to discuss it regardless of whether they

earn more for getting a percentage of their eligible patients into the endos-
copy suite where these procedures are done.

It was with this backdrop that we contemplated how to introduce 4C
as a performance measure to drive quality improvement at contextualizing care. We were mindful that an ever growing number of performance
measures are targeting performance gaps. It also was evident that there
was no countervailing force to the incessant pressure on clinicians to
treat patients with similar demographics and conditions interchange-
ably. What has been missing is a performance improvement strategy for
individualizing care.

In order to harness 4C as a quality improvement strategy we had to
transition from conducting research to implementing quality improvement. In the healthcare field this is often referred to as "translation."
Translating research into practice means taking something that has
been shown to be effective in basic or clinical studies and introducing
it into the actual practice setting so that people can benefit from what
has been learned. We had documented, through our research, that 4C
measures contextualization of care and that contextualization of care
predicts patients' healthcare outcomes. Now we wanted to use 4C as a
performance measure to drive improvement in contextualization of care
and ultimately healthcare outcomes. How to proceed?

The most significant difference between carrying out this work as
quality improvement and as research is that although patients volunteer in both instances, providers cannot opt out of quality improvement.
Participating in quality improvement is not optional. A clinician would
not get far saying to management, "You know, I'm just not comfortable
having you monitor whether my patients are getting colonoscopies so I'd
prefer if you left me out when you collect that data." Allowing providers
to opt out, particularly those with low performance, would undermine
the mission.

In contrast to research, which is monitored by an institutional review
board (IRB), quality improvement projects are monitored by a quality
improvement (QI) committee. Although our colleagues in the research
community are intimately familiar with IRBs, many know relatively little

about how QI committees work or even that they exist. Hence, when we have discussed our work at professional meetings, or submitted manuscripts to publications for peer review, we have heard concerns that by mandating full participation, and without any accountability to an IRB, we are violating ethical norms of human subject research. We find ourselves having to remind our colleagues that they would be right if the participants were still human subjects and we were still researchers. In a QI context, however, they (and we) are employees of an organization just doing our assigned jobs.

Another difference between QI and research is that QI is ongoing. The purpose of a quality improvement initiative is to implement a change that will have a lasting effect on how something is done. Research protocols run for a specified period of time for the purpose of answering a research question. It is possible that knowing that a project is QI and not research may itself be motivating. If providers have the impression that all this audio-recording is just part of some study that will be over soon, it is easy to assume an attitude of "this too shall pass." On the other hand, if they are resigned to the fact that there will be continuous audit and feedback, are shown at regular intervals the errors (and successes) in their performance, and understand that there is no plan to discontinue providing the feedback, then they either have to figure out a way to do better or know that they will continue to see evidence of their subpar performance.

Although physicians are accustomed to all the monitoring, there is a difference between having one's orders or notes reviewed, and actually being audio-recorded while caring for patients. Routine audio-recording of healthcare professionals in the workplace is new. As we embarked on this project, we realized that we had to consider the legal ramifications, the unions to which these providers including the physicians belong, and the perceptions and concerns of the providers themselves.

Early on, we formulated three basic principles to guide the initiative. Each applies to physicians and patients alike. The first was that the project must feel safe. Providers will embrace feedback only if they feel assured that the data does not identify them and could not get them in trouble with management. For patients, we found that the major concern is the potential that it might put their doctors at risk. In addition, they need to feel confident that anything they disclose during a visit is secure and will not somehow be used against them. We planned to use the same encrypted audio devices as we had for the research project, and to explain that we store the data on a secure server space that is certified for housing patient information. The logical way to assure patients that the data would not harm their physicians is to explain how it would be used.

The second principle was to design the project in such a way that it was not an additional work burden for participants. Patients should never be delayed in seeing their doctors because we are holding them up explaining the project in the waiting area. We also agreed to avoid disrupting physicians' workflow. We sought ways to embed the feedback into physicians' regular standing meetings.

The third principle is that the value of the project should be evident to both doctors and their patients. We discovered early on that the best arguments are the real-life examples we compile rather than the quantitative data. Each case that we share to illustrate high or low performance is organized according to the 4C framework: first there is a red flag, then a probe or the absence thereof, then a contextual factor revealed, and then a care plan that is either contextualized or not. A report handed to a small group of physicians with 15 to 20 such examples—and information that all these patients were seen by one of them in the previous month—has a striking immediacy, particularly when the errors are severe. It is hard for anyone to conclude that "this doesn't seem valuable."

Convincing patients of the significance of the project seems to depend on their perceptions of the care they receive. When our team recruits veterans they sometimes respond, "You don't need to look at my doctor here in the general medicine. You should be taping those guys upstairs in the specialty clinics," or " . . . You ought to record those clerks over there . . . the way they treat people!" We emphasize that we are just as interested in collecting data on excellent care as on care with problems.

With these principles as a guide, we began the journey, implementing the project at two sites–Jesse Brown VA Medical Center and Hines Hospital—where we had conducted much of our prior research. We reviewed the audio-recording protocol with the attorney designated to provide legal counsel at these particular facilities. She confirmed that the process was legal as long as veterans volunteered without coercion to carry an audio recorder, and employees were informed that they could be recorded. We also conferred with the facilities' privacy officers, who are responsible for certifying that both clinical and research protocols meet privacy standards for protecting patients' sensitive data. After demonstrating our encryption practices and indicating the server space we use, the project was approved.

At the recommendation of the physician director of ambulatory services at Jesse Brown, our next visit was to the medical center's union stewards to seek their support. We were informed that unions are not authorized to interfere with patient care processes, including quality improvement, as long as the processes do not impact working conditions, such as job duties or employee compensation. We were told, however, that it would be prudent for the union stewards to hear about our project from us first, because a protocol involving concealed audio-recording of employees for whatever reason could spark paranoia and rumor that could undermine the goals of the initiative. We met with the union stewards representing physicians, pharmacists, and social workers and encountered no resistance.

At Hines Hospital we did not meet with the union representatives. We were told that the union representatives are notified of the various official meetings at the hospital, such as meetings of the hospital Quality Council. Two years later, when a union representative complained she had been unaware of the project, we discovered that although her predecessor had attended a meeting at which the project was discussed at its inception, the union had not been notified of Quality Council meetings. Although none of the providers the union was representing had expressed any concerns with the project, we would have liked the union to have been better informed for the same reasons as at Jesse Brown.

When we introduced the project to the physicians we emphasized that this data was for them and them alone. We said, in essence: "We are going to be collecting examples of the best and worst of your care along with metrics on the rate at which you miss contextual red flags and contextual factors, etc., solely for your professional development. If you choose to disregard the data the only ramification is that your patients will continue to get care that is less than optimally tailored to their needs and circumstances, and you will continue to see reports—whether you look at them closely or not—that show the same problems without improvement." As one attending physician put it after seeing a number of the examples from our reports, "Wow, my grandmother could do better than this. She has common sense." That was the kind of response for which we had hoped.

Data collection began uneventfully. Our coders, who took turns handing out the audio recorders and collecting them, were relieved by the simplified protocol, having experienced the project when it was classified as research. No more time was lost waiting for clerical staff to refer patients to them and there was much less paperwork without the consent form documents. Veterans varied substantially in their reactions when invited to audio-record their visits. We continued to back off and discourage participation whenever a veteran seemed reluctant; about 40% of those approached took a recorder into their encounter. But at meetings physicians raised concerns about whether we might be coercing patients, given the suspicions of some of those who participated. We redoubled our efforts to weed out reluctant patients but continued to hear instances in which seemingly enthusiastic veterans subsequently claimed they were recruited to spy.

Our first indication that things might be going pretty well in terms of the feedback came when we presented the first round of data to physicians and other members of the healthcare team at an all-staff meeting at Jesse Brown. We documented that physicians were probing about 40% of the contextual red flags and incorporating about 45% of identified contextual factors into care plans. In other words, in less than half of all cases where there were contextual issues relevant to care planning did we see evidence that these issues were attended to. This would serve as a baseline upon which to improve. Each subsequent report would show a graph, as in Figure 7.1, of both the probing and contextualized plan of care (POC) rate over time, with a summary along the bottom axis of the numbers

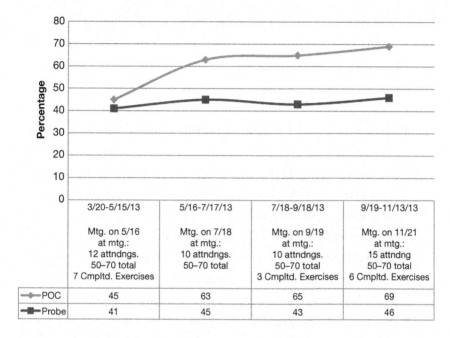

Figure 7.1
Changes in the percentage of contextual red flags that are probed ("Probe") and the percentage of contextual factors addressed in care plans ("POC") at one hospital. Educational interventions and participation levels noted.
Reprinted with permission from reference 2.

of physicians participating in various meetings and other activities we arranged to improve their performance.[2]

Although numbers can be compelling, abstractions like "probe rate" and "contextualized plan of care rate" may not feel meaningful to clinicians. To those of us steeped in the data, they are meaningful because we have seen that they predict patient health care outcomes. More impactful to providers—and more instructive—were the examples we collected. A missed opportunity to contextualize care was presented like this:

Red Flag: The patient missed two appointments that he had scheduled in the past four months.

No Probe: (The physician never asked why.)

Contextual Factor revealed by patient: The patient mentioned that he is having difficulty affording transportation to the VA for his appointments.

No Contextual Plan of Care made: The physician did not acknowledge the patient's comment, nor did he suggest potentially helpful VA services, including travel vouchers available through social services.

Examples showing good attention to context included this one:

Red Flag: Patient mentions he is not using his continuous positive airway pressure (CPAP) machine to protect his heart and lungs from the effects of sleep apnea.
Probe: The physician asks, "Have you tried it?"
Contextual Factor: The patient admits that he has not even opened the package because he heard from a relative that wearing the machine "feels like drowning."
Contextual Plan of Care: The physician explains that although some people feel discomfort with the machine, others feel that it really improves their sleep and how they feel the next day. After some discussion, the patient agrees that he will try the CPAP machine.

Such examples seemed to intrigue many at the meeting because their import is easy to grasp and the presentation of the information is lean. Key elements are extracted from the noise of the visit, revealing a thread of logic or illogic to those providing the care. We spent nearly the entire first hour of a two-hour meeting going over examples. The other half of the meeting dealt with a variety of other well-established performance measures, which fostered a sense of legitimacy and normalcy to our project.

At a second all-staff meeting a couple of months later we handed out case examples to each care team. The meetings took place in a large conference room set up with about a dozen round tables, with each team assigned to a different round table. Examples we selected for this exercise each contained either a failure to probe a contextual red flag or a failure to incorporate a contextual factor into a care plan. Groups at tables were given a few minutes to discuss the case, and then we went around asking each to explain why they thought the clinician overlooked patient context and what they thought could be done differently. As a perk for the physicians, we arranged for them to obtain continuing medical education (CME) credit for participation in the program.

After a few such meetings, spaced a month or more apart, we realized that we needed to up the "dose" of feedback and provide more opportunities for physicians to reflect on what they could do differently to improve contextualization of care. Between meetings we started to send out brief e-mail assignments to physicians, which were designed as reflective exercises based on cases from the prior month. Physicians were reminded that completing these exercises would get them CME credit. It was enough of a carrot that about a third completed all or most of the assignments the first year.

A small number of physicians asked us if we could provide them with individualized feedback based on audio recordings of their encounters only. We always agreed to, but with the caveat that often we had only a small number of audio recordings for any given physician. It was gratifying, however, to see this level of interest. A couple of physicians explained their interest, saying, "I cringe when I see the aggregate data you provide and I'm wondering if I am part of the problem."

During the first 12 months of the project, 2,583 patients across both the Jesse Brown and Hines clinics were approached and invited to participate. Approximately 42% opted in and, of these, 5% were called in to see their doctor before our project staff had finished introducing them to the project and handing them the audio recorder. So, the overall participation rate was 37%. Consequently, we came away with just under 1,000 audio recordings that first year, on about 50 physicians. We noticed signs of what is sometimes called a dose–response relationship, which refers, in this case, to the change in performance of clinicians in response to differing levels of exposure to the educational interventions. For instance, during the first half year at Jesse Brown, we invested a lot of time and effort presenting the data at meetings and engaging providers in various reflective exercises both in face-to-face sessions and online. As illustrated in Figure 7.1, over the first eight months we saw a gratifying improvement in the rate of contextualized care planning from 45% to nearly 70%. That meant that a quarter of the patients whose care depended on addressing factors in their life situation were getting those issues addressed. We started to lose those gains, however, as we diverted our efforts to work on getting the program up and running at Hines Hospital and expanded it to include nonphysician providers, as described below. During the final four months of the first year of the project at Jesse Brown, we were completely absent, except for data collection, and we lost much of our ground; contextualization of care rates fell to 54% by March of 2014.

We observed a similar dose–response relationship at Hines, although the effect was more muted. This may have been, in part, because, for whatever reason, the physicians at Hines started off at a higher baseline level of performance. During the first several months, before we were able to introduce any feedback or organize educational activities, contextualized care plan rates ranged from 54% to 59%, 10 points higher than at Jesse Brown. Furthermore, we had more difficulty getting face time with physician providers at Hines. We went over to Hines repeatedly in the hope of catching physicians at various activities they had planned but met with only a few at a time and often without their full attention. The trend remained flat. Finally, near the start of the second year, we had the opportunity to attend and to have much of the hour at the individual meetings for each care team, just as we had at Jesse Brown. By June of 2014, contextualization of care rates at Hines were at 64%.

Interestingly, while we saw improvement in contextualization of care rates at both Jesse Brown and Hines, we have not yet made much of a dent in the lower of the two lines on our graphs—the probing rate. At both sites it sat between 40% and 45% without budging. What does this mean, particularly when overall contextualization of care rates rise? It signifies that physicians are doing a better job at attending to contextual factors that have already been revealed, but that they are not improving at noticing and asking about (i.e., probing) contextual red flags. In other words, all the feedback and reflection seemed to heighten their responsiveness to the life challenges they already knew about but did not prompt them to investigate for challenges not yet revealed but for which there were clear hints (i.e., contextual red flags). It is possible that a more intensive program of feedback and reflection would have an effect.

EARLY SUCCESS

Here is an example of what successful contextualization sounds like, drawn from our experiences with the VA physicians:

Dr. Harper is seeing Mr. Anderson for a follow-up exam. Dr. Harper runs down the list of medications that Mr. Anderson is on. Mr. Anderson reports that he is taking his blood pressure medication and a medication for his prostate daily as prescribed. Dr. Harper sees that Mr. Anderson also is supposed to be taking a new cholesterol medication, added at the last visit. He asks, "Are you taking the cholesterol medication?" Mr. Anderson replies that he has never taken it.

In the past, Dr. Harper might have written another prescription for the medication and lectured the patient on the importance of following orders. He might have shaken his head and written in the notes, "non-compliant." But this time, he paused. Perhaps it was because he had recently been in a discussion with other providers about patient context, perhaps it was because he had a patient in the past who was not taking his medications because they were being stolen from his mailbox, and Dr. Harper had never guessed that could be a reason for not taking medication. Maybe it was because he felt that he and Mr. Anderson had the kind of relationship where he could probe a little more about his life. Dr. Harper stopped and asked, "Why aren't you taking them?"

Mr. Anderson explained that he had been instructed to cut the pills in half, but he had never received a pill cutter. He went on to say that because he could not cut the pills in half, he did not want to take them incorrectly and so did not take them at all. Dr. Harper was relieved; this was an easy fix. "If I was able to get you a pill cutter, would you take the medication?" "Sure!"

Mr. Anderson received the right treatment at the right time because his physician understood what was going on in his life. His doctor put his care into context.

CONTEXTUALIZATION BY OTHER CLINICIANS AND STAFF

During the first four or five months of the project we only coded data from attending physician–patient encounters. A relatively easy next step was to include residents. The residents who have primary care clinics at Jesse Brown are based in the internal medicine residency program at the University of Illinois at Chicago College of Medicine, and those at Hines are from Stritch School of Medicine at Loyola University. In contrast to the attendings, whom we had to court, the residency programs came to us, because, fortuitously, we offered a solution to a new challenge they faced. The national accreditation organization for internal medicine programs had recently phased in a requirement that all programs incorporate quality improvement activities into their training. Participating in our initiative addressed that requirement.

Introducing an audit and feedback intervention into a residency program is relatively painless because residency programs have routine standing educational meetings and residents are a captive audience. If their residency director wants to do something and it meets an accreditation requirement, they go along with it. That said, the program directors at both institutions had us present the project to their residents and then solicited their feedback. There were some questions, but no one said they did not want to participate. As a next step, we met with the chief residents. The day-to-day educational activities of large residency programs such as these are managed by chiefs who are just one year ahead of the residents in their final year of training. Hence, by engaging and training the chief residents to review and lead feedback exercises on reports, we would no longer need to attend their meetings. We would simply collect and code the data and send them reports.

At Jesse Brown, where we trained the chiefs and attended and observed several of their sessions, contextualized care planning rates increased from 50% to 65% over a roughly nine-month period. As with the QI program for attendings, our efforts at Hines lagged compared with Jesse Brown, largely because the latter is next door to our UIC offices and the former about 10 miles west in a suburb of Chicago. At Hines, where we trained the chiefs at one session but never directly observed them or had them observe us give feedback, performance actually dropped from 61% to 52%. Because there are so many residents and we have so few coders, the sample sizes behind these numbers are too small to approach statistical significance. So these findings should be taken with a grain of salt.

Expanding the project to include nonphysicians introduced a whole new set of challenges. There were several reasons why we held off on adding nurses, pharmacists, and clerical staff. The first is that we did not want to push the envelope: We thought we would see how things went with just physician participation. Second, we wanted to get the other staff familiar with the project before including them. In particular, we were concerned about how their union stewards would react. We thought that if we could tell them that physicians were already participating, and that all other staff were now familiar and comfortable with the project, there would be less chance of pushback. Finally, the 4C coding system had been developed exclusively from analysis of physician–patient encounters, so we would need to figure out how to adapt it to other types of interactions. What, for instance, constitutes a contextual red flag during an encounter between a veteran and a nurse taking vitals, or a veteran and a clerk, prior to a visit?

After one of our presentations at an all-staff team meeting at Jesse Brown, the lead pharmacist approached us and asked if we could include pharmacists in the project. Just getting the request was wonderfully encouraging, because it provided some affirmation that the project was received, at least by some, in exactly the spirit in which it was intended. If pharmacists wanted to be audio-recorded, it meant that they saw value in the data we provide for their own professional development and felt safe that the information was entirely for their benefit.

It was not difficult to add clinical pharmacists because their role at Jesse Brown is in some respects quite similar to that of primary care physicians. Patients seen in primary care who have complex medication management issues, such as from diabetes or high cholesterol, may be referred to a clinical pharmacist for assistance with medication management. So, when a pharmacist sees a veteran who is struggling to manage his or her self-care for a chronic condition, our coding team can look for attention to the same contextual issues–red flags and factors–as those that come up during physician visits.

Soon after, at Jesse Brown, we added nurses and clerical staff. We started by meeting with the supervisors and then with the union stewards. We did not encounter much resistance. Our timing also was fortunate in that patient-centered care of veterans had become the number one priority, coming from leadership nationally. We found that the best way to promote our work was simply to share with people examples of what we were hearing, organized according to the 4C format: contextual red flag, contextual probe, contextual factors, and contextualized care plan.

Once we had support from the unions and managers, we met directly with clerical and nursing staff at their staff meetings. They already knew who we were and what we did. All we had to tell them was that their interactions with patients would similarly be coded and shared for discussion and reflection along with physician encounters. Again, we did not encounter much resistance and even heard rumors of support. The senior nurse manager was particularly enthusiastic.

Including all staff meant that our project team no longer had to restrict participation to veterans in the waiting room who were there to see a physician. If a patient said they were there to see a nurse or a pharmacist, they could now record their visits as well. Adding clerical staff was more of a challenge because it meant intercepting patients as soon as they entered the clinic, before they even got to the front desk, to recruit them and hand them an audio recorder. The LPNs, or licensed practical nurses, who completed the initial intake exam, including checking vitals, had always been recorded, because every patient passes through a nurse's office or station en route to a doctor visit. So, for that group, it was just a matter of coding rather than ignoring the section of each tape that included this encounter.

Our team began listening to these new types of encounters intensively and systematically for the purpose of identifying appropriate contextual red flags and contextual factors. Even when patients check in at the front desk there are opportunities to identify or miss clues that life context is impacting on care. For instance, when patients show up 20 minutes or more late for an appointment, they generally are told they will have to wait until after other patients have been seen (and that the provider will have to approve the late visit). But what if the appointment record indicates the patient has been missing or rescheduling appointments repeatedly? Is the clerk asking the patient if there are any particular barriers to getting to the appointment on time? Might it be, for instance, that another time of day would work better, given the veteran's competing responsibilities, such as a work schedule? We soon learned that clerical staff were taught to follow scripts and policies rather than to think contextually, even though there was often a context to the challenges and concerns veterans brought to the front desk. Hence, at subsequent all-staff meetings, we were able to provide feedback with case examples relevant to everyone with whom veterans interact when they come for a visit.

As the project evolved and new ideas came along, we introduced new features to intensify the feedback. We added a weekly mass e-mail, for instance, addressed directly from our coders to all providers and staff every Tuesday that, alternatingly, summarizes a recent case example of excellent care and a missed opportunity to address and identify context. The goal is to keep the topic on everyone's minds.

In addition to feedback on contextualization of care, our coders wanted to share with care providers or clerical staff observations that did not fit into the 4C system but seemed too important not to disseminate. In the waiting area, they would hear veterans called for their appointment and then passed over or considered late because they were seated in the wrong location, were hard of hearing, or were too slow to get to the desk before others were called. In the exam room, they would hear frequent disruptions as someone knocked on the door to ask the doctor something, or the doctor took a page or answered a phone call in the middle of a discussion with a patient. They noticed that these disruptions sometimes derailed the conversation at a point when the patient was disclosing sensitive information. Some of what they heard was just a startling lack of civility, such as physicians beginning interactions with no greeting or identification. To share these findings, we created an appendix to each report that was printed in blue rather than black font and that gave a variety of examples of things heard on the audio that were critical to patient care but outside of our performance measures. We found these data were often as or more significant in their consequences than the findings in the main report, because what our coders heard and shared was so evidently problematic. It was like holding up a mirror and saying, "Have a look. What do you see?" Responsiveness to the "blue" feedback has been mixed. At all-staff meetings there were discussions about sliding notes under doors rather than knocking on them, but we have not heard of any plans to fix the problems in the waiting area.

To date, we cannot say definitively whether audit and feedback of 4C data works, because we do not have adequate sample sizes and our charge, and hence our focus, has been implementation rather than research. We can only say the trends are favorable, even when the nonphysician providers are added. When we pool data on all staff—clinicians and nonclinicians—at Jesse Brown, where we have had the opportunity to provide the most feedback and facilitate educational interventions, current contextualization of care plan rates hover at about 70%. At this stage, however, when we publish these data it is only to illustrate the process of providing feedback on contextualization of care, rather than to assert that it definitively works. That will have to wait a bit to show. Because we transitioned from research to QI, we have not been prioritizing our project design around answering scientific questions. For instance, in a more scientific design we would find a way to blind our coders so that they do not know whether they are analyzing data from providers who have gotten feedback or from those who have not. The benefit of QI, however, as noted, is that it is the real thing—doctors cannot opt out and it is sanctioned by the institution. We have demonstrated a proof of concept, are monitoring trends, and have a process in place that should be amenable to future study.

OUR FIRST CRISIS

Our move beyond recording only attending physicians also led to our first significant challenge to the QI project. Reviewing a recording, our coders heard an intake nurse, whom we will call Ray Draper, asking a veteran if he was participating in the project. Mr. Draper commented that he did not think government should be spying on people. After this occurred, one of us spoke privately with Mr. Draper to share with him what we had heard and tell him that we would welcome discussing with him any concerns that he had. Initially he asked, "Do I have to participate in this?" and we told him, "Yes," explaining the rationale. We also reiterated how the data is used and not used, particularly stressing that it does not go to a supervisor. We emphasized that if he had any concerns he should not hesitate to talk with us, but never to a patient. It turned out he was relatively new to his job, and it was not clear whether he had attended the all-staff meetings where he would have learned about the project. In any event, at the end of our brief meeting, he emphasized that he was fine with the project and had no concerns. We thought that would be the end of the matter.

Several weeks later, another veteran, who was accompanied by his wife and had agreed to carry an audio recorder, complained to one of our project staff that Mr. Draper denied him access to his doctor's appointment because of his participation in our project. The veteran, whom we will call Roger Meryl, said that after sitting in the waiting area for quite a long time with his hidden audio recorder running, he went up to the front desk to ask about the delay. He was told to talk with Mr. Draper. He went over to Mr. Draper, who said, "I saw you over there talking with that guy with the recorders," pointing to Brendan who was handing out audio recorders that day. "I called you but you didn't respond. That was almost an hour ago." Mr. Meryl's wife, standing next to her husband, asked, "So then why didn't you come over and just get us?" Mr. Draper did not reply.

Mr. Meryl came back to his seat and complained to Brendan, who tried to get the veteran in to see his doctor. The physician was available, but Mr. Meryl was already running late for a back-to-back appointment with another provider, so he had to leave without being seen. Our team followed up with him and his wife over the next several days with several phone calls to get his appointment rescheduled.

When our project group met to discuss what to do, we found ourselves in a quandary. On the one hand, we had emphasized the safety aspect of this project: specifically, that we did not report data to supervisors. On the other hand, this was a serious incident resulting in a veteran not getting care at a scheduled appointment and complaining about it. On top of that, there was a political dimension with ramifications potentially at the highest level. Just several weeks earlier a news story had broken nationally that VA medical centers were not truthfully reporting access problems in their clinics. In the worst example, a clinic in Phoenix had a shadow list of veterans who needed appointments but were kept off the official appointment scheduling system so that it appeared that everybody was seen within a month while, in fact, many waited much longer. The Phoenix incident led to much discussion in Congress, a national investigation of access across the system, and many news stories. This was not the time to risk a news story that a patient had complained about being barred from access, and that we had evidence on tape but that we took no concrete action.

We started by contacting a trusted senior administrator above the level of Mr. Draper's supervisor. We agreed that one of us would attempt one more time to have an informal conversation with the nurse before making an official complaint. Much to our chagrin, however, Mr. Draper was not receptive. Whereas he had seemed friendly and open to cooperation after the first meeting, this time he had no apologies and showed no interest in engaging. He said the problem was that our project team in the waiting area was distracting veterans so that they did not know when they were being called. We pointed out to him that during over 1,000 audio-recorded visits a veteran had never missed a visit because of the QI project, but he was not receptive. We told him that if he could not agree to cease interfering with access, we would have to report the situation to his supervisor. He told us we should do whatever we wanted. Having concluded that we had exhausted other options, we notified the nurse manager. She asked for the audio recorded evidence, so we shared with her the section of the transcript that contained the exchange between the veteran, his wife, and the nurse.

The manager met with Mr. Draper, and because the meeting had potential disciplinary implications, he was invited to include his union representative in accordance with what are called his Weingarten Rights. We never heard a complaint from the union rep, but, nevertheless, a rumor spread that we were using the audio recordings to get people in trouble. The first e-mail came from a physician administrator who had supported the project. Her tone was not happy. She seemed concerned that we had done a bait and switch. She is levelheaded and pragmatic by temperament; all she needed was the facts. When we wrote back explaining the specifics of what occurred, she was entirely reassured and responded that we had done the right thing.

At the next all-staff meeting, after we had finished presenting the latest round of data showing improvements and physician performance and including a number of examples of both excellent practice and missed opportunity, a physician who rarely spoke up at meetings did so. In an angry tone, he said that we were using the project to report staff to their supervisors, and that this was not what he and others had been told would occur. Several other staff chimed in, adding their concern. We explained that the circumstances that led to our report to a supervisor were such that we felt we had no choice and had exhausted other options. In responding, we were cautious about sharing details, given that this was a personnel matter and should not be traceable to a particular individual. Mr. Draper was sitting at a table near the front, the first time we had seen him at a meeting.

We stressed several points. First, that the incident began with a veteran complaining about how he had been treated, not with our responding to something we heard on audiotape. In other words, the audio was used only to corroborate a veteran's complaint. Second, we pointed out that our original promise not to disclose performance data for any participant with their supervisor still held. The information that we disclosed was not performance data. It had nothing to do with contextual red flags or contextual factors. It was evidence of an employee undermining a patient's access to care. Third, we noted that the subject matter of the particular complaint—access to care—was one that the VA could not afford to disregard. Finally, we added that prior to reporting the nurse to a supervisor we had made several attempts to speak with him directly.

Mr. Draper raised his hand and asked who had the transcripts. His voice was calm and matter-of-fact; there was no indication that he was the staff member we were all talking about. Playing along, we replied that the transcripts were in the hands of the supervisor of the individual in question. At that point, the physician who so vociferously opposed the project spoke up saying that he did not think we should have shared the audio transcripts. He said we should have just forwarded on the complaint but without disclosing what was on the audio. At that point Mr. Draper's supervisor, who was also in the room, spoke up defending the project and our reporting of the incident. She said she had the transcripts, that the nurse had not behaved appropriately, and that she discussed it with that person.

We closed by saying we would take the concerns raised to the QI council overseeing the project. The physician who initiated the discussion asked skeptically who was on the council. We mentioned that the council had representation from each of the stakeholder groups. After the meeting, an influential primary care physician who is respected for being evenhanded, helpful, and knowledgeable about how things work in the VA system came over to indicate that he had "no problem" with the project. An advanced practice nurse e-mailed one of us later that morning to say she was concerned, but when we followed up with a phone call and shared the particulars of why we reported the incident, she, too, was supportive. She made the helpful analogy that using audio to corroborate an allegation seems comparable to a surveillance camera corroborating an allegation. Surveillance cameras are not there to spy on employees. They are there for security purposes. But were a veteran to complain that an employee had attacked them in the presence of a camera, there is no reason to think administrators would not or should not look at what was captured on video.

We contacted Deborah Barker, who is director of quality improvement and sits on the QI council. She referred the case to the hospital ethics committee. The director of the ethics committee is a psychiatrist who routinely provides consultation on the care and management of hospitalized patients. Ethicists are often called when a care team, the patient, and/ or their family cannot agree on a care plan. They are accustomed to tense, difficult situations. Our case was distinctly unusual, however, given that it did not involve a particular patient's care. The ethics committee had not been aware of our project and said they knew little about the ramifications of audio-recording staff. They said they would review the case but also wanted a consultation from legal counsel about the incident.

Because the lawyer who had originally approved the project had left, we spoke with another attorney assigned to the VA facility. Legal counsel arrived at essentially the same analogy as the nurse who compared audio to a surveillance camera. The attorney said that we are obligated to report evidence that an employee is "harming" a veteran regardless of whether we see it directly with our eyes or come upon it through the medium of technology. She also pointed out that the use of the transcripts to corroborate the allegations of the veteran was protective of the employee as well as the veteran. We could have just as easily found, from listening to the audio, that the patient's allegations were not substantiated by the audio.

The ethics committee endorsed the opinion of legal counsel. The incident, while unfortunate, brought to the fore the question of when to disclose identifiable data from audio to employees' supervisors. The conclusion of the legal and ethics oversight bodies was that the same standard should apply whether observing misconduct seen in real time or captured inadvertently through technology. Additionally, while ordinarily the tape would be used simply to substantiate or disconfirm a complaint made by a veteran, in egregious, incidentally observed cases

of malfeasance, even in the absence of a complaint, there is a moral obli-
gation to report. Although helpful, the opinion did leave open the question of what constitutes misconduct. We asked the attorney whether she
could identify any specific code of conduct manual for VA employees.
There did not appear to be one. Hence, it is a judgment call. The message
to those wary of being audio-recorded, however, is that the expectations
for good behavior are no different from those in all encounters with
patients.

IS LASTING CHANGE POSSIBLE?

The transition from research to performance improvement has been a
two-year journey, which has not yet answered the question about whether
lasting change is possible. What we have learned from this experience,
however, is that audit and feedback based on audio-recorded data collected by patients for the purpose of improving their care is possible.
There are layers of bureaucracy, legal issues, and general paranoia, but
these are all manageable. One can, in fact, continually assess whether clinicians and care teams are sending their patients home with care plans
that address their individual circumstances and needs.

We can provide feedback based on audio data, but we are less optimistic about whether feedback alone will change anything in the current
health care environment. Until insurance companies, health systems,
the government, or patients themselves say they want to know what is
happening when patients are actually seeking and receiving care, this
work will have limited impact and its support will remain fragile. Not
surprisingly, many are likely to be threatened by this work. The idea that
patients might audio-record physicians or other healthcare professionals
so that a team can evaluate how they are doing can be unsettling to those
professionals. We have persevered, knowing we could get shut down
for an incident such as the one described above—ironic, in our opinion, given who was at fault. We have done our best to protect employees
while giving them the feedback they need to improve, but as the incident

illustrates, there are no certainties they will not get in trouble. Hence, the resistance.

Although we appreciate the importance of protecting employees, what about our duty to patients? If the data are strong—and we think they are—that audio-recordings reveal frequent and serious lapses in the care patients receive, is it not a priority to capture that information and address it? Is improving health care as important as, say, customer service at Comcast? We think so.

In contrast to other performance improvement programs, this one has no carrot or stick. We rely on the commitment of physicians and staff toward self-improvement in the work that they do. As yet, there are neither consequences nor rewards to healthcare teams for continuing to perform poorly or for improving at contextualizing care, respectively.

In the current environment our intervention—the feedback part of audit and feedback—remains quite weak. Regardless, we see a way forward. We have contended with a catch-22—that our transition to QI from research also meant losing the benefits of a more scientific approach. The next step, then, is to return to research with a focus on the feedback piece. We are seeking to use our QI experiences as the foundation for a further set of questions: What is the most effective strategy for providing feedback to clinicians and staff on their performance at contextualizing care that will alter that performance favorably? How high a "dose" of intervention will it take? Does improvement in provider performance yield measurably better health care outcomes and lower costs? Our prior research showed that better contextualization was associated with better outcomes and lower costs, but did not focus on efforts to change any provider's baseline performance. That is not quite the same as showing that *improving* a provider's skills has the same effect. It is a subtle distinction but an important one. Finally, how do participants feel about this work? Are patients really comfortable with what they are doing even when they choose to do it freely? Do providers accommodate over time to assessment with audio as they have to other less intrusive measures of performance? Are managers and administrators invested in driving this sort of change?

Our hope is that others will embrace these questions and help us answer them. We also hope others will join us in this work to see, in particular, if they get the same results. Advancing science depends on demonstrating reproducibility. Regardless of what we find, others will need to arrive at similar conclusions through systematic study to build the foundation of evidence needed to reach a tipping point.

What We Can't Measure
that Matters

"Not everything that can be counted counts, and not everything that counts can be counted."

—WILLIAM BRUCE CAMERON

T he system we developed to help us identify contextualized care, "Content Coding for Contextualization of Care" (4C), identifies lapses in attention to the individual circumstances of a particular patient when those circumstances have evident implications for planning their health care, but it is not particularly nuanced. If we attempted to code more subtle indicators of inattention to context, however, we likely would see considerably more variability in how different coders code the same encounter.

That said, it is worth reflecting on the interactions that are not captured by the 4C coding schema but, nevertheless, have significant implications for contextualized care planning. To gain perspective, it is helpful to consider the clinician–patient encounter as simply two people who are working together to solve a problem, or, at the least, to accomplish something. It is true that in the exam room there is an asymmetry in the relationship: One person is depending on the other, sometimes at a time of great need, and the other is paid to offer those services. The tables, however, could be turned. Let us suppose that instead of being in the exam room, they both are on a busy highway, where the doctor is stranded in the middle of a blizzard and the patient pulls up with his tow truck. Now who is vulnerable and needs help, and who is being paid? There is an asymmetry in every helping relationship that is a function of the immediate circumstance. The two individuals share a common humanity.

Consider the challenge of problem solving with attention to context without the baggage implicit in the "doctor–patient" relationship: It is a cool autumn day, and you are having lunch with Margaret, whom you have not seen for several months. She reached out to you for your advice about whether she should change jobs. She alludes to the fact that she has been encouraged by her boss to leave. You are more senior than she in the industry in which you both work, so your perspective is valuable.

On this particular day, Margaret is uncharacteristically reticent and curt. This is puzzling, because she is the one who suggested getting together. Whereas Margaret is usually animated, even loquacious, today she responds to most questions with a short "yeah" or "not really." Something is not right. Under the circumstances, what would you do? Margaret's change in behavior is a clue that something is going on in her life situation that is affecting her ability to communicate. In 4C lingo, it is a contextual red flag.

You could ignore the behavior, soldiering on through lunch pretending everything is fine. You could attempt to take control: "Margaret, I'm trying to help you and you're not making it easy." You could make an assumption, "I know you must be upset about this change . . ." Or, you could probe, saying, "Margaret, you seem down. Is something bothering you?" This would be a contextual probe to see if you can identify what is going on. You decide to probe.

Margaret responds with, "Sorry. I'm just preoccupied with a lot of work that I need to catch up on. Maybe we should talk more some other time." You are skeptical about her response. Is that really the problem, or is there something else that she does not want to say? In other words, is this a straightforward contextual explanation for her behavior or is there a contextual factor as of yet unidentified? This is where the 4C coding manual instructs coders to give a clinician (or, in this example, the helping friend) the "benefit of the doubt" for a contextual probe. Let us suppose you decide to accept Margaret's claim that competing responsibilities, namely, office work, are the contextual factor, and you respond, "OK, I'm glad it's just that. When you are more caught up on things, just let me know."

In actuality, you have glossed over a number of things. If Margaret is just busy, then why did she not mention it to you at the outset? What about the allusion to her boss wanting her to quit? What, in fact, is the preferred way to respond to Margaret under the circumstances? Her behavior seems mercurial and out of character. It is not all adding up.

What do you do? Do you back off, assuming Margaret is not ready to talk about what is on her mind? Do you push further, sensing that she really does need to talk but is feeling frightened? Or, do you leave it up to her with an open invitation to meet again? The best approach depends, in part, on your level of concern about the situation and your deeper understanding of Margaret's context. If you know, for instance, that Margaret has a history of depression or of making regrettable decisions under stress, you might choose to push a little harder. However, even this decision requires judgment about Margaret's response to such intrusiveness.

One could conceivably apply a 4C model to a microanalysis of every step of the interaction. Although an exchange such as the one above could be assessed for attention to context using the 4C framework, our coders do not actually code so deep. That is because coders do not have adequate information about the nature of the relationship between the two individuals, their prior communication behaviors, or the visual cues that complement speech patterns to make such judgment calls. Yet that does not mean such information is not important. Optimal contextualization of care requires a continuous feedback loop of exploring, processing the information acquired, and responding.

Our system, 4C, is really just a process of coding one cycle, where "exploring" consists of looking for and probing contextual red flags, "processing" is integrating the information acquired to define the problem (i.e., the contextual factor), and "responding" is addressing the contextual factor in a care plan. Telling Margaret you are sorry she is overworked and that you can get together again some other time would be an appropriate plan for a contextual factor, even if there is more under the surface that, if unmasked, would point to a different tactic. Margaret may, in fact, be depressed and feeling unworthy of your attention. Picking up on that requires more than one cycle.

Truly helping people who are feeling vulnerable or are facing complex challenges, or both, involves asking them questions not as an interrogation (which involves, implicitly, looking down at them) but as an act of caring (which sees them eye to eye). In the case of Margaret, it probably involves a carefully calibrated approach to sizing up the situation. For instance, you might say, "I'm sorry you have so much work to deal with. Are things going OK otherwise?" She may respond with tears if she interprets your further questioning of her well-being as permission to open up emotionally. She is assessing whether you are prepared to interlock in dialogue (think of two trains "interlocking" or two hands clasping as they are engaged). At that moment, how you respond will greatly determine whether she pulls back or allows her emotions to well to the surface. If you pull back, she may shut down. You are each modulating the other—you in the caretaker role to signal that you are fully present, she to assess whether you really are. If your intention is to help her solve her problem, whatever it may be, you will not recoil. Rather, you will see her opening up as a small victory and the start of a next cycle of that feedback loop.

WHAT PATIENTS WANT ... (RESPECT)

We have no way to know what proportion of physicians who contextualize care continuously explore, process, and respond with full attention to their patients' needs, but we have a term to describe those who do: engaged. Although, operationally, individuals who engage are aptly described as continuously exploring, processing, and responding to others, such a mechanistic accounting of what engagement entails oversimplifies its essential elements. To engage with others during an encounter is to give them one's full and undivided attention as a fellow human being without preconception about what they are going to say or its implications for subsequent actions.

Engaging represents a complete form of respect. Respect, as we think about it, is fundamentally about regarding others as on level ground—worthy of the same attention we would expect for ourselves. It means not musing about other things while appearing to listen to them, not second guessing what we think they are about to say, not assuming we know what their problems are or what is behind them. In the setting of a medical encounter, it is a sort of cognitive problem-solving mode, with the entire focus on the patient's concerns, needs, and health challenges. An individual who engages will not only perform well when scored using 4C; he or she will go as deep as needed to arrive at the best plan for a particular situation at a particular moment in time. In any given situation, such a person is looking for the optimal next thing to do.

If respect is the underlying impetus for engagement, lack of respect is its impediment—and we think it is the principal one. We are not referring to respect in the narrow sense of admiring others for specific achievements, rather we have in mind the respect that comes from recognition of shared humanity. As our colleague, Simon Auster, often reminds us, we all "urinate, fornicate, and defecate"—strip everything away, and we all share very basic behaviors. A homeless man who stumbles into the doctor's office with strong body odor is just one of us, were we to miss a shower or bath for a few days. Conversely, a characteristic of humanity is that, beyond our bodily functions, we are all unique. Those differences are due to our genetic make-up and the myriad ways in which chance has differentially shaped our lives. From this perspective, it is not hard to respect a homeless man who, living with misfortunes that most of us have been spared, has developed survival skills that few of us have acquired.

In the absence of respect, we are prone to fear others, look down on them, and in nearly all instances, to hold them at a distance. Rather than formulating and asking questions about others' lives, we are filling in the blanks with our own assumptions about their circumstances, or context. In health care, lack of respect can be subtle and hard to detect as we are loathe to recognize it for what it is. Physicians are variously described as detached, aloof, paternalistic, judgmental, and biomedically focused. When we examine the behaviors that inspire these less than desirable adjectives, they have a lack of respect at their core.

The problem of not seeing their shared humanity with patients is evident early in doctors' careers. Recall the medical student in Chapter 1 who, while learning to conduct a medical interview, awkwardly attempted to ignore signs that his patient was distressed (because, it turned out, he urgently needed to make a phone call). Upon observing his attending physician intercede and engage—through exploring, processing, and responding—he exclaimed, "You mean you talk to patients like you talk to people?" What could be more revealing of a lack of respect than not seeing someone as a person?

As this episode illustrates, we may engage with friends—whom we presumably respect as "people"—but keep relationships with patients at arm's length. Many of us treat relationships hierarchically; according different levels of respect based on our perceived status vis-à-vis others. As Margaret loses her composure, would you draw back (i.e., disengage) or lean forward (remain engaged)? We submit that would depend on whether you are able to meet her on level ground. Similarly, we suspect that a physician will more likely disengage from a patient from a lower socioeconomic background than a perceived peer in an emotionally challenging encounter.

Note that regarding others as "on level ground" also applies at the other end of the socioeconomic spectrum. The celebrity who elicits detached awe, a kind of objectification, is not going to receive respectful care. Putting someone on a pedestal is no more respectful than putting them under a pedestal. In either instance, the encounter is not eye to eye. Without the respect, there is a lack of engagement. And without the engagement, the interaction will not uncover and address particular contextual factors, such as lack of privacy, handlers who depend on the celebrity for income, and family dynamics, which may pose challenges to the health and health care of an individual in the public eye.

Although healthcare settings may exacerbate the tendency to objectify or dehumanize others, the extent to which we are able to engage varies even in our personal lives. Some physicians may not engage with their patients because they do not know how to engage with anyone. Like many overachievers, they "manage" everything in their lives, including their relationships with other people—even intimate relationships. The capacity to meet people where they are and to go wherever they need to go is alien to them. They are not familiar with this form of respect. And yet, this is the essential personal quality of the healer.

If you respect someone you will not assume that you know what is best for them, and you will not try to get them to do things your way because you think you know better or that your needs are more important than theirs. If an individual lacks specific competencies, you will intervene to protect them when those deficits threaten their self-interests. A good example is the autonomy of an individual with mild-to-moderate dementia who wishes to continue living alone. If there is a risk this person will leave the stove on and trigger a fire, he should be protected from these potential consequences. Any effort to protect him should be carried out with the goal of preserving his autonomy, so that, as much as possible, he can continue to live in whatever way he chooses. For instance, if his stove were to be replaced with a microwave, he may still be able to live safely at home.

Seeing beyond a person's dementia to elicit her desires and needs, identify her fears, and uphold her dignity requires the full expression of respect. Engaging with an individual with mild-to-moderate dementia means meeting her where she is in conversation, regarding her cognitive deficits as a circumscribed disability but not as a reason to discount her capacity to express her desires, interests, and needs. If the focus of the conversation is her express wish to remain in her home, one attempts to arrive at a care plan that balances her desire for independence with her safety. For instance, one might propose a housekeeper who drops in once a day to help out for an hour or two. Based on the patient's response to various suggestions, one would attempt to maximize her input to arrive at a plan of care that is fully attentive to her context. Such engaged interactions are guided by an appreciation that despite any cognitive limitations, individuals with dementia are still, at a fundamental level, peers in the experience of being human. The desire to choose how we live and to retain dignity—for example, not to be talked down to—is one we all share.

At a basic level, 4C records evidence of engagement or lack thereof. It captures problems when the clinician starts off on the wrong foot, missing obvious cues. Yet it gives full credit too easily. A clinician might initially pick up on a contextual factor and address it based on superficial information but fail to grasp a broader set of issues accessible only through engaged interaction, resulting in a care plan that is ultimately ineffective. For instance, 4C would give full credit for any care plan that attempts to keep the patient with dementia in his home, without discerning between one that is thoughtfully conceived based on the particulars of the patient's life context, and one that might actually increase risk of harm. Statisticians would describe 4C as a specific but not sensitive measure of contextual error. If our coders observe the clinician overlook a contextual factor when planning a patient's care, it is safe to say that the care plan is not appropriate to the patient's needs and circumstances (i.e., there is an identifiable contextual error). On the other hand, we miss a lot of problems with care plans, coding them as appropriate based on one cycle of observation and on our principle of giving clinicians the benefit of the doubt. Hence, physicians who are scored poorly are surely not engaging with patients, as we are unable to document even an initial cycle of exploring, processing, and responding to their patients as individuals. Some of those who perform well are fully engaged, but we do not know how many.

WHAT PROVIDERS NEED ... (BOUNDARY CLARITY)

A common misperception about contextualizing care is that it takes more time than providing algorithmic care that ignores context. As described in our account of work with unannounced standardized patients, we found this not to be true. The same may be said about engagement. Engaging is a way of relating to others and has nothing to do with time. For however much or however little time we have with anyone, we can engage or not.

The perception that engaging is too time-consuming during a clinical encounter reflects on an unfortunate skills deficit: clinicians' inability to set and communicate boundaries. There is nothing inherently disrespectful about telling a patient that the two of you have only 15 minutes together; you are merely relating a fact. Sharing the information is highly collaborative if it is conveyed in the spirit of teamwork, as in, "We only have 15 minutes together, so let's see how much we can get done." Such information gives patients the opportunity to get the most out of an encounter because they can now prioritize their needs. To presume they would be unable to do so is not respectful.

Boundaries here are not defined by the time available for the visit. Boundaries are defined by the separate and distinct needs of the physician and the patient. If engagement is a measure of respect for the other, boundary clarity is a measure of respect for self. Seeing other patients, writing notes, and staying on schedule are things the physician needs to do. When physicians tell their patients how much time they have together and then give their full attention to patients during the available time, there is both boundary clarity and engagement. Patients receive the respect they need and physicians remain mindful of their own needs. When the physician does not set boundaries, the lack of clarity serves neither's interests. The physician is chronically "running behind" and feeling anxious, and the patient has a distracted physician.

It is common for us to hear medical students and residents say, "I couldn't get him to stop talking." or "I was afraid to ask because I know he'll go on and on." or "I really didn't want to be rude and interrupt, so the visit went way over." The sense of helplessness they describe characterizes difficulty with recognizing boundaries. It is not their job to control whether the patient is talking or not. That is up to the patient. It is their job, however, to guide the visit such that the patient has the best opportunity to get the most out of it. We have yet to see a patient take offense when a physician interjected either to propose that he could better assist the patient if more attention were spent on something else or simply to let her know he had another patient to see. The former might be accomplished with, "I'm sorry to cut you off, but we only have a few minutes left and there are some other things I would like to help you with before the visit is over." The reason patients, in our experience, are not generally offended (although they may be frustrated with the system) is because there is, in fact, nothing offensive about telling someone how you think you can best help them or what your needs are. When physicians are unclear about their own boundaries, they avoid asking questions that—as some colleagues have put it—"open a Pandora's box" for which they have found "there just isn't time." Such guardedness precludes engagement. Hence, without boundary clarity, clinicians will not readily engage.

Boundary clarity is about more than being able to manage the time constraints during a visit. It is about appreciating the boundary that separates people as autonomous individuals. Hence, a lack of interpersonal boundary clarity interferes with listening and observing in encounters with others because one is not able to distinguish between the information that is coming in and one's reaction to it. There is a blurring of sense of self with sense of other.

Consider again your lunch with Margaret. Let us suppose her reticence made you think, "What am I doing to make her mad at me?" or "She is being rude. I am insulted ..." or "I'm boring her." Would you realize that these are reactions coming from you rather than information sent by her? If you cannot distinguish the two, then you are not able to explore, process, or respond to her behavior effectively. Sorting out the contextual factors in Margaret's life that account for her behavior becomes difficult because of the extraneous information that is coming from you but that you think is coming from her. When you are able to make that distinction, it signifies clarity about the boundary that separates you from others. Note, the goal here is not to do away with certain emotions but to recognize them for what they are. The fact that you take things personally that are not personal is OK, as long as you understand that is what is happening. An absence of such boundary clarity elicits in the clinician a tendency to be judgmental as a defense against perceived slight. Rather than recognizing that the angry patient is depressed, the physician who concludes he has been insulted becomes either defensive or distant, in the latter instance disengaging and—as quickly as possible—"putting the lid" back on the box.

In addition to trouble managing boundaries, another likely reason for the perception that engagement diminishes the efficiency of the visit is that engaging requires forfeiting control over the agenda of an encounter. It is not possible to engage if one is intent on telling another person what they need to do. Patients are unlikely to follow through on instructions if their perspectives, concerns, and priorities are not addressed. Hence, a doctor-driven agenda may feel efficient to the doctor who can now check off a lot of boxes on her "to do list," but little if anything is accomplished that benefits the patient. On the other hand, if the same interaction is engaged, the physician may not make much headway on her "to do list," but she enlists the patient as a partner in care planning. In the long-term, the benefit to the patient is much greater.

A capacity to allow an encounter to go where the patient needs it to go, such that the most important contextual red flags emerge, is another competency 4C cannot measure. We only are able to assess the performance of clinicians at addressing the issues that have an opportunity to percolate to the surface under the terms of a visit, or that are evident in the medical record. And given how poorly many clinicians perform at recognizing and addressing these most basic challenges, we surmise that what we are measuring is the tip of a large iceberg.

ELEMENTS OF A HEALING RELATIONSHIP ...
(ENGAGEMENT WITH BOUNDARY CLARITY)

Engagement and boundary clarity are, in a sense, both opposed and interdependent. Attempting to engage with others without boundary clarity is a recipe for chaos and harm. When angry spouses are yelling at each other in an all-out fight, each has the other's full and undivided attention, the interaction is unselfconscious, gloves are off, and each person is on level ground. What is missing is respect—specifically respect for personal boundaries. They are likely "pushing each other's buttons," which, in turn, triggers each to react to their own emotional responses rather than to the content of what is said. Hence, while they think they are responding to each other, they are actually responding to something coming from within. Neither is clear about "what is me" and "what is you." The boundary line is gone, so each is crossing into the other's space. When there are boundary violations during an interaction, there is heat without light. Time passes, much is said, but little is heard. Two people are engaged in a fight but not in a productive encounter.

At the other extreme, people might hold each other at such a distance that there can be no engagement. The interaction is, literally, "impersonal" in that the personhoods of the two individuals are not able to come into contact. Imagine our couple now so disengaged that they do not discuss issues that are affecting them other than essential activities of daily living, such as shared child care responsibilities or who will do chores. Neither of them is getting their deeper concerns addressed. Instead of loud heated arguments, there is now a chilly interaction. In the exam room, this most often is because the physician is holding the patient at arm's length. He or she addresses the patient formally, is polite, but inscrutable. The patient has no idea what the physician is like as a person. What the care provider has done, in essence, is put nearly everything about herself that is distinct off-limits. The patient does not have access to a real person to engage with and is, therefore, limited in what he can or will communicate. One cannot engage with someone playing a role. One can only engage with a person who is fully present.

Of the two extremes, our experience is that doctors err much more often on the side of holding patients at a distance, such that their personal boundaries do not come into contact. They are considerably more social than the prototype of the inscrutable physician described above, but their approach is nevertheless highly socialized. As one colleague put it, "My patients are not my friends." Interestingly, she is someone whose patients probably like her. She has taken one of those medical communication courses and tries to follow what she has learned, beginning with "setting the stage" for the visit (also called "building rapport"), eliciting information, giving information, understanding the patient, and ending the encounter—five steps in a well-known medical communication curriculum with the acronym "SEGUE."[1] No doubt—or one can surmise at least—when she is communicating with friends she does not follow a communication task list. The fact that physicians have to learn to communicate with patients in the first place says a lot. Presumably the vast majority of them know how to communicate with friends and family (although that is an untested assumption). The paradox is that medical communication courses reinforce the paradigm that physicians need to learn to communicate from someplace that is not the place where they, as unique individuals, generally reside. They are learning to communicate from a contrived persona. If they master that persona, they may convince their patients that they are who they appear to be.

Such a manner of relating to patients has been well described and endorsed by the mainstream medical establishment. Clinicians interested in physician–patient communication have looked outside of the medical field to the service industry and to research on human relations. A paper on the topic, published in *JAMA: The Journal of the American Medical Association*,[2] proposed that physicians conduct "emotional labor," which they described as involving two types of acting: surface acting, in which the provider "forges empathic behavior" and deep acting, in which they "generate empathy-consistent emotional and cognitive reactions." The authors state that both of these have been adopted successfully "by service workers, such as flight attendants and bill collectors" but are not yet widely appreciated in medicine. But on close examination, it becomes clear that these are no more than techniques to achieve an impersonal goal: A repeat customer, a calmed passenger, a debt recovered. The practitioners—certainly the bill collector—would just as soon not be recognized as individuals by those they are serving. Whatever their usefulness, such techniques hardly serve to elevate the clinical encounter above the routine and hardly increase regard for the patient as more than a carrier of disease, to be treated according to an algorithm.

Doctors are not the only ones who keep a distance to avoid engagement. Patients will do this, too. And the effect is similar. The human being who is the patient is inaccessible, rendering attention to context in care planning minimal. A recent extreme example illustrates the challenge.

When one opens David Mason's chart, a "behavioral warning flag" pops up that reads, "Mr. Mason has had multiple incidents of verbal and physical abuse of staff and other patients; he also made a serious threat against staff. Avoid caring for the patient in secluded areas. If Veteran does not respond to de-escalation and verbal redirection by staff, call VA police." Mr. Mason, who is 56 years old and six feet tall, has been coming to the Jesse Brown VA Medical Center since 1996. He recently became one of our patients after a previous doctor refused to care for him any longer. The final straw was that the patient was angry the physician would not prescribe narcotics and, in a visit to the emergency room to try to get the medication, he mentioned that he could kill his doctor for not giving him what he needed. The ER informed the physician of the incident. The physician said he would not see the patient again.

What is most striking about reviewing the 2,724 notes written about Mr. Mason over nearly 20 years, is how little information is contained within them. Among hundreds of notes by primary care physicians, social workers, psychiatrists, and case managers, among others, we find just a few facts about his life, typically cut-and-pasted from one record to the next. We see that he was born and raised in Chicago and lived with four sisters and two parents. His dad suffered from depression and alcoholism. A note mentions that for a part of his childhood he was sent south of the city to live with a grandmother to keep him out of reach of gangs. He finished the 11th grade, served in the Marines for just one year, with no combat exposure, and then left with an honorable discharge after a training accident on an obstacle course resulted in a herniated disc. For about eight years, he worked in maintenance for the Chicago Housing Authority. His life since has been chaotic, with two failed marriages, domestic abuse, alcoholism, snorting cocaine, two prison terms for burglary, and a couple of suicide attempts with pill overdoses. Many of these life events are documented in real time as they played out during his years coming to Jesse Brown VA Medical Center. Perusing through thousands of notes, one catches fragments of things as they occur. His first prison term, for instance, is registered as a two and a half year gap in the chart. He did not come in for visits, and the first note upon his return simply says he was away in prison.

New hardships have hit. He lost all three of his adult children. A 26-year-old daughter was raped and murdered the prior summer. Before that, a 37-year-old daughter died of an overdose. A 21-year-old son was shot and killed. Most recently, he had a heart attack followed by three-vessel coronary artery bypass graft surgery (CABG) that was performed at an outside VA hospital.

Three VA police officers were called to stand by as Mr. Mason was led into the exam room. They stood outside with their bulletproof vests, noisy walkie-talkies, and pistols as an attending physician and a resident shut the door to the exam room. After introducing himself and the resident, the attending leads the way:

"Mr. Mason, I'm sorry to have the police just outside the door but I understand from the chart that you've threatened people and there is a notice saying we have to have the police stand by. I also understand that you've been frustrated about other doctors not giving you narcotics for your pain. Can you tell me about the pain you are having?"

The opener is markedly direct. The elephant in the room is named: that there are police guarding the two physicians and that the patient has a particular demand. Airing these observations takes some of the wind out of Mr. Mason's sails. Before Mr. Mason has a chance to play out his script, the doctor is saying, "Yes, I know you intimidate your doctor and make demands," and then following this comment immediately with an undeniable request of his own. How can Mr. Mason not answer the question, "Tell me about your pain?" if he is demanding narcotics? The attending is sitting just a couple of feet away from the veteran and looks and feels interested and relaxed.

Mr. Mason ignores the question and launches into a litany of complaints about VA doctors not helping him get the Norco that he needs.

The attending replies that he would like to help him out with any medical issues, including pain, but that there are several reasons he will not prescribe a narcotic. The first is that he sees from the record that the patient has had cocaine show up in several urine drug tests. To prescribe narcotics to a patient who is using cocaine is considered dangerous, and as a physician, he could lose his medical license for doing that. He is not prepared to take that risk. Second, he sees that for months while Mr. Mason was getting prescribed narcotics, his urine did not have any narcotics in it—just cocaine—which indicates he was not taking the prescribed drug anyway.

The patient replies, "Doc, I know I've made mistakes, but I'm in pain and you've got to help me. My last two urine tests have been cocaine-free." The physician replies, "Show me where it's hurting," and pulls closer to the patient. Mr. Mason points to several areas including his back, his hand, and a leg. The physician examines each body part, taking the veteran's hand in his as he looks and gently pokes at the areas that he is told hurt. While he examines Mr. Mason, he asks him questions about how long he has had these pains. Then he asks him where he lives, and Mr. Mason says he is homeless. He says he avoids shelters because they are violent and dirty, preferring to sleep outdoors. They talk about some of the places where he is able to stay safe and warm. The physician comments that upon reviewing the medical chart, he saw that a social worker, who has been following Mr. Mason's case, has noted that they seem very close to getting him housed through a special program for homeless veterans. The doctor asks Mr. Mason, "How optimistic are you that this is all going to work out in the next couple of weeks?" Mr. Mason replies, "I'm really not convinced." The doctor says, "Let's see if we can reach the social worker," and picks up the phone. There is no answer, so he leaves a message. He also sends an e-mail.

During the visit, the conversation expands. Mr. Mason brings up the deaths of his three adult children. He talks about his remorse that he has been such a bad example to his family. He describes how his grief at the death of his children is compounded by guilt and says that he is trying to provide good care to his grandchildren, for whom he now has a lot of responsibility. They are scattered about, but he says that he keeps a close eye on them, and notes that when he is housed he will become more involved. What stands out during the conversation is the coherence of Mr. Mason's thought processes and use of language. He does not say things that are unnecessary or tangential. His responses to questions are concise. He speaks using sentence structure correctly. He is open about himself and direct. All of these are marks of intelligence, and the attending points that out. He says to Mr. Mason, "You know, one thing I notice about you is that you are obviously intelligent. Actually, very intelligent." Mr. Mason nods quietly, accepting the compliment with a simple, "Thank you." He has probably not been told that in a while. He may not think about his intelligence often, but he also probably knows that he is smart. Maybe he senses the lost potential. The attending turns to the resident and asks aloud, "Do you know how I could tell he's intelligent?" The resident stares back blankly. The attending points out how the ways a patient communicates are tip-offs. Mr. Mason sits there looking mildly intrigued.

As the attending wraps up the encounter, Mr. Mason demands narcotics again. The interaction had been going well and was headed for a tidy closure on what might be interpreted as the physician's terms, at least in Mr. Mason's mind. As he saw the end of the visit approaching, he acted as though someone had thrown a switch. Calm thoughtful discussion switched to indignation, agitation, and a demanding rant that if he could not have narcotics there was no point being there. He said he would have to get himself another doctor. He looked hurt and angry. However, he never seemed threatening. He got up and stormed out. The attending noted, however, a slight reluctance in his gait as he left, suggesting that something about the encounter made him ambivalent about leaving. His behavior seemed a bit theatrical.

A few weeks later, Mr. Mason showed up for a follow-up visit. This time the team called for just a single officer. The attending greeted Mr. Mason in the waiting area and ushered him back into the exam room. He noticed an interesting feeling in himself. Whereas he had felt a certain sense of dread awaiting the encounter, as soon as he saw Mr. Mason and began to interact with him, that dread was replaced with a good feeling, a feeling that this man could engage with him. The visit would have substance.

It started out with the expected demand for medications. The doctor already had ascertained that this was Mr. Mason's way of asserting control in a world and setting where he otherwise felt helpless. The demands get him attention and derail other agendas. It is striking how completely they have crowded everything else out, as evidenced in his medical record. Mr. Mason has diabetes for which he takes medications, yet no one has checked a HgB A1c in two years; he has heart disease, yet no one has checked his lipids. Mr. Mason has successfully kept his doctors at arm's length. More specifically, he managed to ensure that they keep him at arm's length. He does not know how else to protect himself. He is prone to becoming vulnerable to others, so he works hard to avoid that happening. He subverts the possibility of engagement not by holding others at a distance, but by threatening others' boundaries so that, instead, they hold him at a distance.

This time, however, he has a problem. The new doctor is not responding as expected. He is not keeping Mr. Mason at arm's length. Interacting with his new physician requires engaging, an opportunity that is seductive, but fear holds him back. Mr. Mason does not trust anyone, particularly physicians.

The doctor embraces the good feeling he has toward Mr. Mason and again sits comfortably facing him. He says he remembers the housing issue and wonders how that is going. Mr. Mason replies that he now has an apartment and that this is a big relief. He says it does not have much furnishing or bedding, however, and he is having trouble getting clean and insect-free secondhand items. They discuss the places he has tried, including the Salvation Army and a VA basement warehouse that serves homeless veterans. During the conversation, Mr. Mason mentions that although he is glad to be housed, the grief he feels at the loss of his children and the mistakes he has made go with him everywhere, whether on the streets or in an apartment. Because he wants to be there for his grandkids, he does not feel he is at risk of hurting himself. The doctor says he is concerned about Mr. Mason's diabetes and his heart condition and would like to discuss those and see what they can do. Mr. Mason returns to his cry for narcotics. Again, that switch has flipped. He says there is no point staying if he cannot get Norco and that he needs another doctor. He gets up and exits. The attending wonders, as he watches Mr. Mason stumble out, whether he is running away from something he fears. He looks vulnerable.

Reviewing his chart, the doctor notices an interesting pattern: Although Mr. Mason has led a life of intimidation, there is no documentation that he has actually hurt anyone. Three long-term relationships with women play themselves out in the medical record over the span of two decades. Two of the women came to appointments with him, both apparently spouses for a few years. There is mention of his putting his hands around their necks or, in one case, threatening to light his wife on fire while she is asleep, but he is the one who tells these stories, not they. It is also clear that he has been victimized a few times, including suffering stab wounds. Mr. Mason is a big guy and imposing, but it is not clear he is violent. He may be, but the proof is not there. Interestingly, he denies one of the charges that landed him in jail, a burglary he says he did not commit. The other one, which occurred when he was younger, he does not deny. That one was 18 years ago.

A week later, the doctor calls Mr. Mason at his new apartment to see how he is doing. Another man answers the phone. He says Mr. Mason is busy with a couple of his grandkids. When he is told Mr. Mason's doctor is calling, the man says to wait a minute, that he will come to the phone. Mr. Mason picks up the phone and he and his doctor talk for a few minutes. It is not a good connection. The call is dropped twice, requiring call-backs. Mr. Mason says he has gotten some bedding and winter clothing, but he is not convinced it is clean, so he is soaking it in his tub. He still needs a good pair of boots because there has been snow. He cannot stay on the phone long as he says he is watching several kids. There are voices in the background. They end the call.

Will Mr. Mason come back? If he does, will he begin to attend to his health needs, particularly his diabetes and heart disease? His last two urine toxicology screens have been negative. Can he continue to avoid cocaine? Is the death of his third child—his 26-year-old daughter just seven months earlier—and the ensuing responsibility of his grandchildren a point of grief and responsibility that will mobilize him to function as a caretaker? Who else is involved in their care? How old are they? And are they at risk of abuse or neglect?

To find out the answers to these questions and, potentially, to influence the course Mr. Mason's life takes, the attending will need an engaged relationship. He will continue to reach out to Mr. Mason with an occasional brief call, a checking-in, so to speak. The outcome will depend on Mr. Mason's capacity for trust. He has learned he cannot scare his doctor away through demands that make other physicians feel guilty and uncomfortable, trigger hostile interactions, and justify his storming out. In truth, his beseeching does make his new doctor feel badly—reminding him of the power imbalance implicit in his authority to dispense a powerful medication—but he neutralizes that imbalance by reminding his patient that he, too, is accountable. Were he to misuse his power there would be consequences for him as well. In essence, the doctor's refusal to look down on him is yet another confounder to Mr. Mason's attempts to play to the insecurities and ego needs of his physicians, such that they hold him at a distance while he gets the attention, albeit negative, that he craves. "This guy's different," he may be thinking or sensing. "He's calling me at home. I can't push him away."

There are two possible outcomes: If Mr. Mason is prepared to stay in touch—with the ensuing vulnerability that entails—he will enter into a therapeutic relationship with his physician that is grounded in two people working together to solve problems as equals. On the other hand, if trusting others whom he cannot control is not an option, he will do what he can to extract himself from this budding relationship. He will find himself another doctor. Although the latter may be more likely, the VA will not make it easy for him. If he tries to switch physicians again, he will learn that veterans are only allowed to do that once a year at Jesse Brown. Because his prior physician was the one who severed the relationship he might be allowed to switch again, but the VA would discourage his doing so without good reason. Reflecting on the the rule the doctor smiled to himself and thought, "Mr. Mason may be stuck with me." He appreciates that his patient's best hope is to have a rock he can grab hold of or at least periodically return to—if he is able—for some stability and perspective in an otherwise chaotic life. That is the doctor's contextualized plan of care. It is not a plan, however, for which we know how to give credit.

Bringing Context Back Into Care

Do not study what disease the patient has; study what patient has the disease.
—Sir William Osler (attrib.)

A technician can be defined as one who knows every aspect of his job–except its ultimate purpose and social consequences.
—Sir Richard W. Livingston (attrib.)

We have a long way to go before patients can realistically expect that the care they receive is right for them—that it takes into account the particular challenges and needs in their lives at that time. The journey to contextualized care and patient-centered decision-making has just begun. To briefly review where we have been, here is what we know:

- Every patient is an individual, and many face life situations that make guideline-based medicine inappropriate.
- Care that is not tailored to patients' lives is more costly and less beneficial.
- Doctors do a poor job of identifying these life situations, and even when they do, they do not always know how to incorporate them into plans of care.
- If we want to improve (or even correctly measure) these skills, we have to directly observe providers taking care of patients in their

natural environment—to look behind the white curtain and beyond the medical record.

We hope we have convinced you that we have documented a deep and difficult problem in the healthcare system. The problem is prevalent, serious, and not detectable using the usual tools of medical chart review. Characterizing and exposing this problem has been a major focus of our research.

How should the world respond to the evidence that attending to patients' individual needs and circumstances helps them resolve many of the challenges to managing their illnesses? In some respects, we hope that it would be with a big yawn. Few scientists aspire to bore their audience with the obviousness of their findings, but in our case there is a certain logic to that aspiration. First of all, if people can agree that attending to patients' individual needs in care planning—contextualizing their care—is self-evident, and that we have simply cast a light on it so that the evident becomes visible, then we can begin to talk about how to make the most out of the instruments we have developed for shining that light. Second, although we hope to bore people with our findings so that we can move on to applying them, we do not expect anyone will be bored with the methods for making these discoveries. The strategies for directly observing care through concealed audio recording, whether by unannounced standardized patients (USPs) or actual patients, cry out for much more curiosity and experimentation.

At social events, when we tell people we meet about the work we do, they are intrigued by the espionage but not generally surprised by our findings. Often they are prompted to tell us stories of incidents they or their family members have experienced in which physicians were unhelpful. Some of these anecdotes are perfect examples of contextual error. (Others simply illustrate poor communication or uncaring behavior.) Conversely, they tell us about great care they received, again sometimes due to a physician picking up on an important contextual clue. We do not pretend to have cornered the market on defining all that is good and bad in the doctor–patient relationship. Our focus in these studies is on a specific cognitive process, or its lack.

Our peers can be a harder sell, and while we appreciate intellectual skepticism, it can be frustrating. We welcome the peer review process that determines publication or funding when it works to challenge us to discover problems or unrecognized limitations in the work that we do. But sometimes we wish reviewers themselves would think harder, particularly when critiquing a new and potentially transformative area. On the one hand, there are those who say, "This work is nothing new. People have been studying the doctor–patient relationship, patient-centered communication, the importance of picking up on cues, and the essential value of empathy for years." True. But they have not rigorously defined these terms in a way that can be operationalized to discern whether specific cognitive tasks are accomplished during a visit. The broad subject area in which we work probably has its origins in the phrase, "the art of medicine." The term "art" has perhaps contributed to an unfortunate perspective that what we are so concerned about is precious but unmeasurable. It is what medical students often referred to as "the touchy-feely" part of their training, where it is OK to tune out a bit in class. We are still struggling to convince people to turn their brain back on when looking at our work; and to challenge us with hard questions grounded in the data we produce, rather than dismiss the work based on assumptions that they have seen it all before. We really do not think they have.

On the other hand, we have colleagues who look at our study design with the rigor of experimental scientists but without consideration for the unique subject matter and setting. We have been told that our work cannot be taken seriously until we do a randomized controlled trial of contextualization of care. Randomized controlled trials, or RCTs for short, are considered the gold standard for experimental design. We are practiced at RCTs. We adopted that design to assess whether an educational intervention improves performance at contextualization of care, as we discussed in Chapter 6. But what we have not done is assign patients randomly to receive care that is contextualized or explicitly not contextualized. Doing so seems unethical. Imagine asking patients to agree to a study in which there is a 50% chance that their doctors will intentionally recommend care that is not appropriate to their needs and circumstances. When reviewers say they would like to see this sort of data, we do not think that they are proposing an unethical study design. We think they just are not thinking. Fortunately, enough of our peers fall into neither of these groups, enabling our work to see daylight in a variety of publications, and reach a diverse audience.

In addition to laypeople and researchers, there are the clinicians. Clinicians are less likely to question the data, but unless they have personally participated in either our research or quality improvement project (which we discussed in Chapter 7), they are apt to react with suspicion to the whole endeavor as yet another "big brother" tactic. This is understandable. Who would not question a proposal to have their work covertly audio-recorded? We later describe in detail the strategies we have adopted to address these suspicions and fears.

Finally, healthcare administrators are quick to anticipate how doctors will react, which provokes their anxiety about the fallout and backlash that could occur with a program of concealed audio-recording. When assured that it works great as long as you have clinicians' buy-in, they, too, split into two camps: those who think it is terrific because it could improve care, and those who see it as a low priority because regulators do not mandate this level of scrutiny and they certainly will not reimburse for it. Both are right. With respect to the latter, until Medicare takes the lead in calling for data based on directly observing the clinical encounter—either via USPs or real patient volunteers—it will not likely be coming to a doctor's office near you.

As detailed in Chapter 8, throughout this project we have had an ongoing awareness that while we are making significant strides in measuring effective physician–patient communication and decision-making there is much that we are not capturing. The emphasis of our work has been on building a foundation that includes new concepts and terms, along with new tools of measurement, and then on applying and refining them to demonstrate how they are useful. But it is only a foundation. We are aware that there is more to attending to context in healing interactions than what we are documenting or assessing at this stage. But we regard the concepts and terms described in this book as essential to conceptualizing more nuanced variations in how healthcare providers—or anyone in a healing role—attend to subtle clues about context during interactions. We are not convinced, however, that there are practical ways to measure those variations.

Of course, there is a lot of work left to do. We know how we would like doctors to think about patients and how we would like them to behave as care providers. Although we have had some success in improving physician knowledge, skill, and performance in contextualizing care through education and feedback programs, a wholesale re-emphasis on patient-centered care will require a concerted and coordinated effort at many levels. Although there are more research questions we would like to answer, we also think the time is right to move the importance of contextualized care out of the purely academic realm and into the mainstream of care.

HOSPITALS AND PROVIDERS

We appreciate the effort and resources expended to try to build systems for providing health care that put the patient at the center—medical homes and (at the VA) patient-aligned care teams. We are frustrated, however, by what appears to be a failure to grasp the underlying problem, which is a lack of engagement between healthcare providers and the patients for whom they care. When two people are engaged, one will notice when the other seems to be struggling with something and will ask him or her about it.

Physicians blame technology, lack of time with patients, reimbursement policies, etc. for not engaging. These system factors certainly do not encourage engagement, but engagement occurs in the moment, anywhere, and under almost any circumstances. It happens when people are open to one another, take a genuine interest in each other, manifest curiosity, and, in healing relationships, try to help someone else overcome a challenge or solve a problem. As discussed in Chapter 2, when physicians take the time to figure out what is really going on with patients, they make it up by avoiding wasted effort going down the wrong path. Their visits are not, on average, any longer. Until that engaged attention to patients is the organizing principle for patient-centeredness, new approaches and processes for care delivery will never fulfill their intended promise.

Is engaged attention to others a specialized skill that is no longer the purview of the busy doctor? Compare it to microscopy, for instance, which revolutionized the practice of medicine by enabling physicians to examine the composition of blood and tissue, and to use the number, type, and form of the cells they saw to diagnose disease and guide treatment. Not every physician is adept with a microscope, and people trained specifically in laboratory work have largely supplanted the microscope in each doctor's office. If preventing contextual error saves money and improves health, might there be a role for professional contextualizers on the healthcare team—especially skilled in talking with patients and discovering life context relevant to their care?

Both nurses and patient advocates have the potential to fill this role, at least partially, and help patients by bringing context to the attention of physicians. There are organizations that contract with employers and payers to provide telephone health assistants who aid clients (employees and members) with healthcare and claims needs. Some of these health assistants are nurses; many are not. When we applied the 4C coding method to telephone calls between clients and health assistants in one such organization, we found that the health assistants' clients were more likely to reveal their life context spontaneously during the call, but also that health assistants were substantially better at probing and incorporating context into their assistance than physicians usually are. In part, this may be because helping clients understand how their medical needs interact with the rest of their lives in order to receive the right care is a core mission of these health assistants.

In hospitals and other large practice settings, adding contextualizers to the healthcare team might be an important complement to physician-centered strategies, but will never substitute for the presence of these skills in physicians themselves. It is one thing to outsource looking into a microscope to identify microbes, but another thing entirely for physicians to ask others to see their patients in all their complexity so that they do not have to do so. Attending to the particular needs and circumstances of individuals when planning their care must be a core competency of clinical practice. Testing for contextualization skills when recruiting physicians, and implementing programs to help them develop and master these skills, not only would address a healthcare quality problem but also send a message to medical educators that they are not consistently turning out the professionals that patients need.

PAYERS AND REGULATORS

The healthcare system comprises not only doctors and other care providers, but also the systems of delivery, payment, and regulation. In the United States, physicians must comply with licensing and practice regulations established by state medical boards. In order to receive payment for their care of the majority of patients, they must follow rules established by insurance companies and state and federal governments.

In addition to regulations (what doctors can do and what doctors must do), healthcare delivery is increasingly characterized by the use of incentives to physicians who achieve performance targets for their patients. For example, a part of a physician's salary may depend on what portion of his patients with diabetes have received a foot exam, or how many women patients have had a screening mammography by age 55. These "pay for performance" incentives seek to motivate physicians to order tests or prescribe treatments that are known to be beneficial for most patients but are underused. But such incentives are also insensitive to patient life context, rewarding the recommended care whether or not it is the most appropriate care for a particular patient. This is not unlike rewarding the prescription of amoxicillin for urinary tract infections even when it is not appropriate for a particular individual. For most patients, it is inexpensive and highly effective; for the patient allergic to penicillin (or the woman taking birth control pills, which become less effective when taken with amoxicillin), it could be a serious error.

We are of the view that the quality improvement movement in health care has not yet grasped the seriousness of overlooking patients' circumstances and needs in care planning. In all fairness, we are the only researchers that we know of evaluating performance in this area, and measuring its impact on outcomes and costs—one reason we would like to see others take on this work as well. Until there is a broad appreciation that it is just as important to tailor care to patients' individual needs and circumstances as it is to ensure that it is based on the best research evidence, there will not be improvement. Changes in attitudes take time. Fifteen years ago, when performance measures were phased in to evaluate physician attention to research evidence, there was a lot of resistance. Physicians complained their autonomy was infringed upon. However, the evidence that physicians were not providing the standard of care became so widespread that a tipping point arrived, favoring conventional performance measures. That tipping point is still a ways off for tracking contextualization of care.

A regular program of direct observation (especially by unannounced standardized patients) and performance feedback could be a much more effective measurement and enhancement of good care. One day, such programs might be adopted as regulatory requirements, or could serve as the basis for more nuanced incentives to reward physicians not only for recommending the standard care beneficial for the average patient but for recommending alternatives when patient context dictates that the standard care will be ineffective. In the meantime, practices and providers might be encouraged by their payers to adopt direct observation programs on their own both as a competitive advantage in the marketplace and a way to control costs while providing better and more patient-oriented care.

MEDICAL EDUCATORS

We are both medical educators, and we naturally wonder about whether and how medical education has contributed to physicians' propensity for contextual error, and whether and how it can instead develop patient-centered decision-making skills.

Traditional medical education in the United States begins before medical school, as college students prepare to take the Medical College Admission Test (MCAT). Until 2015, that meant spending a lot of time studying biology, chemistry, and physics; consequently, most "pre-med" students were science majors. The test—and, as a result, medical schools—favored those whose focus was on the biomedical rather than the psychosocial. Beginning in 2015, however, the MCAT includes a major section on the psychological and social foundations of behavior, including topics that mirror several of our contextual domains, such as access to care, attitudes toward illness, and cultural beliefs. We have yet to see the impact of these changes on new medical school applicants, but they are likely to shift the focus of college education to emphasize a better understanding of context.

As we mentioned in Chapter 6, medical schools try to round out their applicants by conducting interviews rather than relying solely on test scores. In particular, schools have adopted the "multiple mini-interview" (MMI) format, in which students are asked to respond to several short "stations" designed to assess humanism, professionalism, moral reasoning, and other "non-cognitive" qualities not easily evaluated by MCAT scores.[1] Although these assessments are a good way to predict performance in medical school, we have argued that contextualization is not just empathy or humanism. We do not yet know whether or how well contextualization skill can be predicted from these kinds of interviews; based on the performance of current medical students, however, we expect the answer is "not very well."

There is no question that medical students can be attuned to the importance of patient context; our randomized trial discussed earlier in this book, in Chapter 6, demonstrated that even a relatively short course can lead to measurable improvement in competence at contextualization. One way to try to make these improvements translate into future performance is to make the focus on patient contextualization ongoing and habitual, rather than a one-time course with a one-time test of skill. This will require ongoing supervised interactions with patients (or unannounced standardized patients) in the clinical setting. As anyone who receives care at a teaching hospital knows, medical students are often the first providers in the exam room who ask the patient to explain their problem and its history; the students later present their findings to the resident or attending physician. The training students receive in taking and presenting a history is an important part of their medical school experience, and one that easily could be enhanced by a continual focus on probing patient context and its impact on health and health care. Students are already taught to form a differential diagnosis of possible medical explanations for the patient's symptoms; they should simultaneously be forming a contextual differential diagnosis of life circumstances that may underlie or contribute to the symptoms or pose barriers to their resolution. The six axes introduced in Chapter 5 might also serve a useful learning function for doctors-in-training.

If medical schools need to make contextual thinking a habit, residency programs need to reinforce that habit and deepen the understanding of context within the resident's specialty. Residents have much more responsibility than medical students in the management of patients, and should be particularly attuned to the need to incorporate contextual factors into care plans. Nearly all of our work has focused on general internal medicine, one of the broadest of medical specialties, and although much of what we learned will apply to other specialties, each may have unique contextual issues that can only be appreciated through engagement with patients. Pediatrics and psychiatry, in particular, may require an even broader consideration of life context.

Once out of residency training, physicians may be licensed to practice in their respective states and are eligible to take a specialty board exam and become "board-certified." Board-certified physicians are required to regularly maintain their certification through a combination of repeat testing, continuing education and self-assessment, and engagement in practice-improvement programs. This maintenance of certification (MOC) process offers a great chance to employ direct observation approaches to improve contextualization of care. Unlike many practice improvement programs, directly observed care does not require extra time or steps during the patient exam—the physician does exactly what he or she normally does with patients. The improvement comes when the unique data that can only be obtained through direct observation allows the physician to reflect critically on practice, learn about missed opportunities to probe and incorporate patient context, and develop and try out new ways to engage with patients. We are currently working with the American College of Physicians in a pilot project using unannounced standardized patients as part of such a performance improvement program.

PATIENTS

Do patients have a role in preventing contextual errors? On one hand, we have seen over and over in our research that when patients take the initiative to tell about the challenges they face, to "hit their doctor over the head with it" rather than waiting or hoping to be asked, they are more likely to get the care they need. And because we know that it is less likely for physicians to incorporate contextual factors they have not themselves probed, astute patients who present their context also need to be vigilant in reviewing the care plan—subjecting it to a "reality check" based on their context.

Several books have suggested techniques for patients to make sure that their doctor hears their needs. Some of these books describe in great (if anecdotal) detail how doctors miss clues and make reasoning errors. The books then recommend that patients work to keep their doctors from making these mistakes, for example, by bringing in a written history, asking the doctor key questions, and taking notes during the visit. There is a lot of value to these techniques, although some of them are more difficult to accomplish during an acute illness. Indeed, working with VA investigators, we are helping to test a context checklist that patients could fill out before their visits to help their physicians remember to ask about potential red flags. Patients who are fortunate enough to have a choice of doctors also might think about how their doctor would chart on the six axes we describe in Chapter 5, and if they are not happy with the picture, consider another provider.

On the other hand, patients themselves often do not know what is important in their care and how their context may interfere. The asthma patient who has lost his health insurance and is using his daily steroid inhaler only when he is having symptoms may not understand that the inhaler will not be effective. His doctor would. He also may not know that a cheaper generic version of his name-brand inhaler may be available. His doctor should. He may assume that the doctor already knows about his life situation, or that everything is recorded (correctly) in the medical record. It is not. And he may be intimidated by the difference in status between himself and his doctor. ("She doesn't want to hear about my problems with my job, she's too busy and important.")

Most of us would hate to meet with a lawyer knowing we were responsible for making sure she gave good legal advice and catching what she missed. Patients should be aware that doctors can make contextual errors, and do their best to recognize when doctors are off track, but they are not likely to fix this problem by thinking like doctors for them.

By being more explicit about their needs and challenges, patients can partially—but only partially—offset the shortcomings of clinicians functioning as technicians rather than engaged professionals. As patients, we rely on our doctor to think about how a particular surgery will limit our capacity to meet our particular life obligations, and then share that information with us. Just as contextualizing care cannot entirely be outsourced to nonclinicians, it also cannot be outsourced to the recipients of care. It is a fundamental attribute of the healer. That is why it is essential to address in the education and assessment of those upon whom we depend when we need care.

NOTES

PRELIMS
1. D. Osborne & T. Gaebler. *Reinventing Government: How the Entrepreneurial Spirit is Transforming the Public Sector*: Addison-Wesley Publishing Company. Boston, MA; 1992.

CHAPTER 1
1. Roter, D., & Larson, S. (2002). The Roter interaction analysis system (RIAS): utility and flexibility for analysis of medical interactions. *Patient Education and Counseling, 46*(4), 243–251.
2. Ross, L. (1977). The intuitive psychologist and his shortcomings: Distortions in the attribution process. *Advances in Experimental Social Psychology, 10*, 173–220.
3. Weiner, S. J. (2004). Contextualizing medical decisions to individualize care: lessons from the qualitative sciences. *J Gen Intern Med, 19*, 281–285.
4. Weiner, S. J. (2004). When something is missing from the resident's presentation. *Academic Medicine, 79*(1), 101.

CHAPTER 2
1. Field, M. J. & Lohr, K. N. (1990). *Clinical practice guidelines: Directions for a new program* (Vol. 90). Washington, DC: National Academies Press.
2. Steinberg, E., Greenfield, S., Mancher, M., Wolman, D. M., & Graham, R. (2011). *Clinical practice guidelines we can trust.* Washington, DC: National Academies Press.
3. Kohn, L. T., Corrigan, J., & Donaldson, M. S. (2000). *To err is human: Building a safer health system.* Washington, DC: National Academies Press.
4. Reason, J. (1990). *Human error.* Cambridge University Press. Cambridge, England.
5. Rosenhan, D. L. (1973). On being sane in insane places. *Science, 179*, 250–258.
6. Dresselhaus, T., Luck, J., & Peabody, J. (2002). The ethical problem of false positives: A prospective evaluation of physician reporting in the medical record. *Journal of Medical Ethics, 28*(5), 291–294.

7. Glassman, P. A., Luck, J., O'Gara, E. M., & Peabody, J. W. (2000). Using standardized patients to measure quality: Evidence from the literature and a prospective study. *The Joint Commission Journal on Quality and Patient Safety.26*, 644–653.
8. Luck, J. & Peabody, J. W. (2002). Using standardised patients to measure physicians' practice: validation study using audio recordings. *BMJ, 325*(7366), 679.
9. Luck, J., Peabody, J. W., Dresselhaus, T. R., Lee, M., & Glassman, P. (2000). How well does chart abstraction measure quality? A prospective comparison of standardized patients with the medical record. *The American Journal of Medicine,108*(8), 642–649.
10. Peabody, J. W., Luck, J., Glassman, P., Dresselhaus, T. R., & Lee, M. (2000). Comparison of vignettes, standardized patients, and chart abstraction: A prospective validation study of 3 methods for measuring quality. *JAMA: Journal of the American Medical Association, 283*(13), 1715–1722.
11. Green, A. R., Carney, D. R., Pallin, D. J., Ngo, L. H., Raymond, K. L., Iezzoni, L. I., & Banaji, M. R. (2007). Implicit bias among physicians and its prediction of thrombolysis decisions for black and white patients. *Journal of General Internal Medicine, 22*(9), 1231–1238.
12. Weiner, S. J., Schwartz, A., Weaver, F. M., Goldberg, J, Yudkowsky, R., Sharma, G., ... Abrams, R. I. (2010). Contextual errors and failures in individualizing patient care: A multicenter study. *Annals of Internal Medicine, 153*(2), 69–75.
13. LaCombe, M. A. (2010). Contextual errors. *Annals of Internal Medicine, 153*(2), 126–127.
14. Graham, J. (2010, July 19). Mystery patients' help uncover medical errors. *Chicago Tribune.*
15. Schwartz, A., Weiner, S. J., & Weaver, F., Yudkowsky, R., Sharma, G., Binns-Calvey, A., Preyss, B., & Jordan, N. (2012, July 7). Uncharted territory: measuring costs of diagnostic errors outside the medical record. *BMJ Quality & Safety.*

CHAPTER 3
1. Weiner, S. J. (2012). *Content coding for contextualization of care coding manual.* Retrieved from http://hdl.handle.net/1902.1/19356.
2. Schwartz, A., Weiner, S. J., Binns-Calvey, A. & Weaver, F. M. (2015). Providers contextualise care more often when they discover patient context by asking: meta-analysis of three primary data sets. *BMJ Quality & Safety.*

CHAPTER 4
1. Weiner, S. J. (2012). *Content coding for contextualization of care coding manual.* Retrieved from http://hdl.handle.net/1902.1/19356.
2. Schwartz, A., Weiner, S. J., Binns-Calvey, A. & Weaver, F. M. (2015). Providers contextualise care more often when they discover patient context by asking: meta-analysis of three primary data sets. *BMJ Quality & Safety.*

CHAPTER 5
1. Bazeley, P. (2013). *Qualitative data analysis with NVIVO* (2nd ed.). Thousand Oaks, CA: Sage Publications.

2. Gawande, A. (2010) *The checklist manifesto: how to get things right* (1st ed.). New York: Metropolitan Books.

3. Bloom, B. S. (1956). *Taxonomy of educational objectives; the classification of educational goals* (1st ed.). New York,: Longmans, Green.

4. Graber, M. L., Franklin, N., & Gordon, R. (2005). Diagnostic error in internal medicine. *Archives of Internal Medicine, 165*, 1493–1499.

CHAPTER 6

1. Weiner, S. J. (2004). From research evidence to context: the challenge of individualizing care. *ACP Journal Club, 141*, A11–A12.

2. Weiner, S. J., Barnet, B., Cheng, T. L., & Daaleman, T. P. (2005). Processes for effective communication in primary care. *Annals of Internal Medicine, 142*, 709–714.

3. Weiner, S. J. (2004). Contextualizing medical decisions to individualize care: lessons from the qualitative sciences. *Journal of General Internal Medicine, 19*, 281–285.

4. Schwartz, A., Weiner, S. J., Harris, I. B., & Binns-Calvey, A. (2010). An educational intervention for contextualizing patient care and medical students' abilities to probe for contextual issues in simulated patients. *JAMA: Journal of the American Medical Association, 304*, 1191–1197.

CHAPTER 7

1. Asch, S. M., McGlynn, E. A., Hogan, M. M., Hayward, R. A., Shekelle, P., Rubenstein, L., . . . Kerr, E. A. (2004). Comparison of quality of care for patients in the Veterans Health Administration and patients in a national sample. *Annals of Internal Medicine*, 141(12):938–945.

2. Weiner, S. J., Schwartz, A., Sharma, G. (2015). Binns-Calvey, A., Ashley, N., Kelly, B., & Weaver, F. M. Field notes: Patient collected audio for performance assessment of the clinical encounter. *The Joint Commission Journal on Quality and Patient Safety*, 42(6):273–278.

CHAPTER 8

1. Makoul, G. (2001). The SEGUE Framework for teaching and assessing communication skills. *Patient education and counseling*, 45(1):23–34.

2. Larson, E. B., & Yao, X. (2005). Clinical empathy as emotional labor in the patient-physician relationship. *JAMA: The Journal of the American Medical Association*, 293(9):1100–1106.

CHAPTER 9

1. Reiter, H. I., Eva, K. W., Rosenfeld, J., & Norman, G. R. (2007). Multiple mini-interviews predict clerkship and licensing examination performance. *Medical Education, 41*(4), 378–384.

BIBLIOGRAPHY

Asch, S. M., McGlynn, E. A., Hogan, M. M., Hayward, R. A., Shekelle, P., Rubenstein, L., . . . Kerr, E. A. (2004). Comparison of quality of care for patients in the Veterans Health Administration and patients in a national sample. *Annals of Internal Medicine, 141*(12), 938–945.

Bazeley, P. (2013). *Qualitative data analysis with NVIVO* (2nd ed.). Thousand Oaks, CA: Sage Publications.

Bloom, B. S. (1956). *Taxonomy of educational objectives; the classification of educational goals* (1st ed.). New York: Longmans, Green.

Dresselhaus, T., Luck, J., & Peabody, J. (2002). The ethical problem of false positives: a prospective evaluation of physician reporting in the medical record. *Journal of Medical Ethics, 28*(5), 291–294.

Field, M. J., & Lohr, K. N. (1990). *Clinical practice guidelines: Directions for a new program* (Vol. 90). Washington, DC: National Academies Press.

Gawande, A. (2010) *The checklist manifesto: how to get things right* (1st ed.) New York: Metropolitan Books.

Glassman, P. A., Luck, J., O'Gara, E. M., & Peabody, J. W. (2000). Using standardized patients to measure quality: Evidence from the literature and a prospective study. *Joint Commission Journal on Quality and Patient Safety, 26,* 644–653.

Graber, M. L., Franklin, N, & Gordon, R. (2005). Diagnostic error in internal medicine. *Archives of Internal Medicine, 165,* 1493–1499.

Graham J. (2010, July 19). Mystery patients help uncover medical errors. *Chicago Tribune.*

Green, A. R., Carney, D. R., Pallin, D. J., Ngo, L. H., Raymond, K. L., Iezzoni, L. I., & Banaji, M. R. (2007). Implicit bias among physicians and its prediction of thrombolysis decisions for black and white patients. *Journal of General Internal Medicine, 22*(9), 1231–1238.

Kohn, L. T., Corrigan, J., & Donaldson, M. S. (2000). *To err is human: building a safer health system.* Washington, DC: National Academies Press.

LaCombe, M. A. (2010). Contextual errors. *Annals of Internal Medicine, 153*(2), 126–127.

Larson, E. B., & Yao, X. (2005). Clinical empathy as emotional labor in the patient-physician relationship. *JAMA: Journal of the American Medical Association, 293*(9), 1100–1106.

Luck J., Peabody, J. W., Dresselhaus, T. R., Lee, M., & Glassman, P. (2000). How well does chart abstraction measure quality? A prospective comparison of standardized patients with the medical record. *The American Journal of Medicine, 108*(8), 642–649.

Luck, J., & Peabody, J. W. (2002). Using standardised patients to measure physicians' practice: validation study using audio recordings. *BMJ, 325*(7366), 679.

Makoul, G. (2001). The SEGUE Framework for teaching and assessing communication skills. *Patient education and counseling, 45*(1), 23–34.

Osborne, D., & Gaebler, T. (1992). *Reinventing government: How the entrepreneurial spirit is transforming the public sector*: Addison-Wesley Publishing Company, Boston, MA.

Peabody, J. W., Luck, J., Glassman, P., Dresselhaus, T. R., & Lee, M. (2000). Comparison of vignettes, standardized patients, and chart abstraction: a prospective validation study of 3 methods for measuring quality. *JAMA: Journal of the American Medical Association, 283*(13), 1715–1722.

Reason, J. (1990). *Human error.* Cambridge University Press. Cambridge, England.

Reiter, H. I., Eva, K. W., Rosenfeld, J., & Norman, G. R. (2007). Multiple mini-interviews predict clerkship and licensing examination performance. *Medical Education, 41*(4), 378–384.

Rosenhan, D. L. (1973). On being sane in insane places. *Science, 179,* 250–258.

Ross, L. (1977). The intuitive psychologist and his shortcomings: Distortions in the attribution process. *Advances in Experimental Social Psychology, 10,* 173–220.

Roter, D, & Larson, S. (2002). The Roter interaction analysis system (RIAS): utility and flexibility for analysis of medical interactions. *Patient Education and Counseling, 46*(4), 243–251.

Schwartz, A., Weiner, S. J., Harris, I. B., & Binns-Calvey, A. (2010). An educational intervention for contextualizing patient care and medical students' abilities to probe for contextual issues in simulated patients. *JAMA: Journal of the American Medical Association, 304,* 1191–1197.

Schwartz, A, Weiner, S. J., Weaver F, Yudkowsky, R., Sharma, G., Binns-Calvey, A., . . . Jordan, N. (2012, July 7). Uncharted territory: measuring costs of diagnostic errors outside the medical record. *BMJ Quality & Safety.*

Steinberg, E., Greenfield S., Mancher M., Wolman D. M., & Graham, R. (2011). *Clinical practice guidelines we can trust.* Washington, DC: National Academies Press.

Weiner, S. J., Barnet, B., Cheng, T. L., & Daaleman, T. P. (2005). Processes for effective communication in primary care. *Annals of Internal Medicine, 142,* 709–714.

Weiner, S. J., Schwartz, A., Sharma, G., Binns-Calvey, A., Ashley, N., Kelly, B., & Weaver, F. M. (in press). Field notes: Patient collected audio for performance assessment of the clinical encounter. *The Joint Commission Journal on Quality and Patient Safety.*

Weiner, S. J., Schwartz, A., Weaver, F. M., Goldberg, J., Yudkowsky, R., Sharma, G., . . . Abrams, R. I. (2010). Contextual errors and failures in individualizing patient care: A multicenter study. *Annals of Internal Medicine, 153*(2), 69–75.

Weiner, S. J. (2012). Content coding for contextualization of care coding manual. Retrieved from http://hdl.handle.net/1902.1/19356.

Weiner, S. J. (2004). Contextualizing medical decisions to individualize care: lessons from the qualitative sciences. *Journal of General Internal Medicine, 19*, 281–285.

Weiner, S. J. (2004). From research evidence to context: the challenge of individualizing care. *American College of Physicians J Club, 141*, A11–A12.

Weiner, S. J. (2004). When something is missing from the resident's presentation. *Academic Medicine, 79*(1), 101.

Page numbers followed by "f" and "t" indicate figures and tables.

4C. *See* Content Coding for
    Contextualization of Care

Access to care, as domain of patient
    context, 17, 89
Acting, emotional labor and, 177
Actors, 41–43, 63. *See also* Standardized
    patients; Unannounced standardized
    patients
Actual patients. *See* Real patients
Administrators, 189
American Board of Internal
    Medicine, 123
American Medical Association
    (AMA), 45–46
Analysis, 107, 107f
Anti-social behavior, 10–11
Application, 107, 107f
Art of medicine, 188
Ashley, Naomi, 63
Assessment. *See* Performance measures
Assumptions, 169–170
Attitude toward illness, 17, 89
Audio recordings. *See* Recordings
Audit and feedback process, 137
Auster, Simon, 84, 169

Autonomy, 171
Awareness Principle, 83
Axes differentiating physicians
    contextual vs. noncontextual thinkers,
        116–117
    distractibility vs. multitasking
        capability, 114–116
    flexible vs. rigid interactions and,
        101–105
    overview of, 101, 117–119, 118f
    premature closure vs
        open-mindedness, 109-112
    systems reviewing vs. theory building
        approach to taking histories,
        105–109
    timing of planning care and, 112–114

Backchanneling, 97
Bandwagons, xviii
Barker, Deborah, 161
Bedside manner, 115
Benefit of the doubt, 167
Bentham, Sheila, 20–22
Bias, real patients and, 69–70
Billing, 53. *See also* Costs
Binns-Calvey, Amy, 42–43, 62–63

Biomedically-focused care. *See also*
    Standardized care
  context missing from, 17–20
  contextual errors and, 28–31
  elements missing from, 3–5
  faulting the patient and, 10–13
  high costs of, 13–17
  history of, 26–28
  inattention to context and, 5–8
  physician decision-making and, 8–10
  standard training process and, 121–123
  unannounced standardized patients
    and, 31–39
Biomedical reasoning, 123
Blame, assigning to patients, 10–13
Blinders to context, 5–8
Bloom's taxonomy of learning objectives,
    107, 107f
"Blue" feedback, 156
Board-certified physicians, 195–196
Boundary clarity
  engagement and, 175–185
  respect and, 172–175
Breakfasts, 64–65

Care deferrers, 112–114
Care planning, timing of initiating,
    112–114
Carter, Jennifer, 11–12
Cataloging, 96–97
Catch-22, 163
Change, lasting
  assessment of, 136–140
  early success and, 151–152
  likelihood of, 162–164
  overview of, xxi
  process improvement and, 140–151
  workshops and, 135–136
The Checklist Manifesto (Gawande), 106
Checklists, 106, 108, 114
Christoff, Eric, 52
Clarity. *See* Boundary clarity
Cleanup, 43–44
Clerical staff, 154–156
Clinical education, 122

Clinical expertise, 125–126
Clinical Performance Center, 64
Clinical practice guidelines (CPG), 27. *See
    also* Guidelines
Clinical reminders, 141
Clinical state, 125
CME. *See* Continuing medical
    education
Coding
  complete process, 89–90
  guidelines for addressing contextual
    factors, 85–88
  guidelines for exploration of contextual
    factors, 82–85
Cohn, Barry, 6–7
Communication behaviors, cataloging
    of, 96–97
Communication boundaries. *See*
    Boundary clarity
Competence, performance vs.,
    134–136, 135t
Competing responsibilities, 17, 89
Complications, 36, 49–50, 50t
Comprehension, 107, 107f
Computerized Patient Records System
    (CPRS), 115
Computers, 114–116. *See also*
    Distractibility
Content analysis software, 100
Content Coding for Contextualization of
    Care (4C)
  coding exploration of contextual
    factors and, 82–85
  coding management of contextual
    factors and, 85–88
  crisis and, 157–162
  outcomes and, 89–90
  overview of, 66–69, 68f, xx–xxi
  as performance measure, 140, 142
  perspective and illustration of, 79–82
  physicians at Jesse Brown VA Medical
    Center and Hines Hospital and,
    140–151
  rationale for development of,
    76–79, 97–98

residents, pharmacists, nurses, clerical
    staff and, 152–157
Roter Interaction Analysis Scale
    vs., 97–100
use of to answer tough
    questions, 90–91
Context, 5–8, 17–18
Contextual differential, 16–17, 129, 195
Contextual errors
economic costs of, 53–56, 56f
overview of, 28–31
real patients and, 69, 74–75
unannounced standardized patients
    and, 37–39, 50–51, 50t
Contextual factors
coding physician exploration of, 82–85
coding whether physicians are
    addressing, 85–88
Contextualized plan of care rate,
    146–147, 147f
Contextualizing care
defined, xiv, xvii
early success and, 151–152
engagement and, 20–22
requirements of, 17–20
research on, 23–24
teaching, 123–131
Contextual probing, 67, 82–83, 146–147,
    147f, 150–151
Contextual red flags, 80–82. See also
    Red flags
Contextual thinkers, 116–117
Continuing medical education
    (CME), 149
Control, engagement and, 175
Cookie-cutter medicine, 139–140
Corner Bakery breakfasts, 64–65
Costs. See also Billing
of caring for fake patients, 46
(economic) of contextual errors,
    53–56, 56f
reducing by contextualizing
    care, 13–17
Council on Ethics and Judicial Affairs
    (CEJA), 45–46

CPG. See Clinical practice guidelines
CPRS. See Computerized Patient
    Records System
Creation, 107, 107f
Critical thinking, importance of,
    107–108
Cultural/spiritual beliefs, 17, 89

Davis, Melanie, 10–11
Dawson, Thelma, 14–17
Deception, 41
Decision-making
differential diagnosis and, 129
examining the mundane and, 8–10
lack of teaching for, 125
patient-centered, 126–127, 127f
Deep acting, 177
Degrees, 122
Dehumanization, 170
"Demanding" label, 11–12
Dental care, 86–87
Dentist avoidance, 12–13
Differential diagnosis, 129
Directly-observed care, 139–140,
    189, 193
Distractibility, 114–116
Doctor-centered utterances, 98
Doctoring, xvi–xvii. See also Humanistic
    medicine
Dose-response relationships, 149–150
Draper, Ray, 157–162

EBM. See Evidence-based medicine
Education. See Teaching
Edward J. Stemmler, MD Medical
    Education Research Fund
    grants, 132
Eisen, Seth, 47
Electronic medical records, 43–44,
    114–115
Emails about fake vs. real patients, 46–47
Emotional labor, 177
Emotional state, 17, 89
Empathic socioemotional exchanges, 98
Encryption, 43

Engagement
  boundary clarity and, 175–185
  importance of, 20–22
  overview of, xviii
  respect and, 168–172
Environment, 17, 89
Errors. *See* Contextual errors;
    Medical errors
Errors of execution, 29
Errors of planning, 29
Ethics committees, 161
Ethics review committees. *See*
    Institutional Review Boards
Evaluation, 107, 107f
Evidence-based medicine (EBM), 26–27,
    125–127, xv, xviii
Execution errors, 29
Exploring, 167

Face time, 51
Factorial design, 37, 37t
Feedback, 141, 149, 156
Financial situation, 17, 89
Flexible interactions, 101, 103–104, 105
Fundamental attribution error, 10, 25

Garcia, Amelia, 3–6, 10, 13, 129–130
Gates, Eli, 11–13
Gawande, Atul, 106
Gideon, Patrick, 13–14
Graham Clinical Performance Center, 41
Grants, 132
Guidelines, xv–xvi. *See also* Clinical
    practice guidelines

Hand-shaking, 10–11
Harris, Ilene, 124
Haynes, Brian, 127
Hidden recorders. *See* Recordings
Hierarchies, relationships and, 170
Hines Hospital, 144–157
HIPAA (Health Insurance Portability and
    Accountability Act of 1996), 49, 65
Histories, approach to taking, 105–112
Holloway, Don, 80–82, 85–86

Hospitals, 190–192. *See also Specific
    hospitals*
Human Error (Reason), 28
Humanistic medicine, xv, xvi–xvii
Hypoglycemia, 110

Incentives, 192–193
Insensitivity, 8–9
Institute of Medicine (IOM), 27, 28
Institutional Review Boards (IRB)
  lasting change and, 142
  real patients and, 60, 64
  unannounced standardized patients
    and, 40–41
Insurance, 33, 52
Interaction analysis, 98–99
Inter-rater reliability, 68–69
Interrupting, 8–9
Interviews, 121

IRB. *See* Institutional Review Boards
Jesse Brown VA Medical Center, 48, 141,
    144–157, 178–179
*The Journal of the American Medical
    Association* (JAMA), 134, 177

Kamin, Carol, 96
Kelly, Brendan, 63

LaCombe, Michael, 52
Lasting change. *See* Change, lasting
Learning objectives, 107, 107f
Legal concerns of recordings, 143–145
Legitimizing, 98
Loyola University, 152

Maintenance of certification (MOC), 196
Mason, David, 178–185
MCAT. *See* Medical College
    Admission Test
Medical College Admission Test (MCAT),
    121, 194
Medical Decision Making, 125
Medical errors, 27–28, 49–51, 50t
Medical record review, 30

Medical records, 33
Medical school, 122–123, 124–125,
    194–196. *See also* Training
Mehta, Suresh, 12
Memorization, 107, 107f
Meryl, Roger, 157–158
Metrics. *See* Performance measures
Miller, George, 135
Miller's Pyramid, 135
Minimal competency, 79
Misuse of medical resources, 55–56
MMI. *See* Multiple Mini
    Interview format
MOC. *See* Maintenance of certification
Model probes, 82–83
Multiple Mini Interview (MMI) format,
    121, 194
Multitasking capability, 114–116
Murawsky, Jeff, 48–49
Mystery patients, 32–33, 34. *See also*
    Unannounced standardized patients

National Board of Medical
    Examiners, 132
National Institute for Health and Care
    Excellence (NICE), 27
National Patient Care Database (VA), 44
Needles, fear of, 12–13
NICE. *See* National Institute for Health
    and Care Excellence
Nodes, NVivo program and, 100
Nonadherence, 6
Noncompliance, 5–6
Noncontextual thinkers, 116–117
Nurses, 154–156, 191
NVivo program, 100

Objectification, 170
Open-ended psychosocial questioning, 98
Open-mindedness, 109–110
Outcome measures, 138–139
Overuse of medical resources, 54–56

Patient advocates, 191
Patient-centered care, 98, xv

Patient-centered decision making,
    126–127, 127f
Patient-centered utterances, 98
Patient context, 126–131, 127f. *See also*
    Context
Patient preference, 126
Patients, 10–13, 168–172, 196–197. *See*
    also Real patients; Unannounced
    standardized patients
Patient satisfaction surveys, 30–31
Pattern recognition, 110
"Pay for performance" incentives, 192–193
Performance, competence vs., 134–136, 135t
Performance incentives, 192–193
Performance measures
    overview of, 138–140
    process improvement and, 140–151
    for science and safety, xv
Performance pay goals, 141
Pharmacists, 153–156
Phoenix VA Hospital, 158
Physicians
    boundary clarity and, 172–175
    engagement and, 168–172
    prevention of contextual errors and,
        190–192
    real patients and, 61, 64–65
    standard training of in U.S., 121–123
Planning errors, 29
Preclinical education, 122
Premature closure, 109–110, 113
Preventative Services Task Force, 27
Probe rate, 146–147, 147f, 150–151. *See*
    also Contextual probing
Process improvement, 140–151
Processing, 167
Process measures, 138
Providers, 190–192. See also *Specific*
    providers
Pseudopatients. *See* Unannounced
    standardized patients

Qualitative methods, 124
Quality improvement, 140–151, 156–157,
    162–163, 193

Quality improvement (QI) committees,
    142–143, 160–161

Race, 39, 51, 52
Randomized controlled trials (RCT),
    188–189
Rapport building, 176
Real patients. *See also* Unannounced
    standardized patients
    advantages of use of, 60t
    overview of study using, 58–70, xix–xx
    results of study using, 70–75, 73f, 74f
Reason, James, 28
Recorders, 43
Recordings
    legal issues of, 143–145
    overview of, 33, xix–xx
    performance measures and, 140
    real patients and, 59, 65–66
    selection of, 42–43
    unannounced standardized patients
        and, 40
Red flag outcomes, 90
Red flags. *See also* Contextual red flags
    Content Coding for Contextualization
        of Care and, 67–69, 68f
    real patients and, 66–67, 71–72
    unannounced standardized patients
        and, 36–37, 50–51
Regulators, 192–193
Relationships, hierarchy and, 170
Relationship with healthcare
    providers, 17, 89
Research evidence, 125–126
Residency programs, 122–123, 152–157
Respect
    boundary clarity and, 172–175
    engagement and, 168–172
Responding, 167
Review of systems (ROS), 106
RIAS. *See* Roter Interaction Analysis Scale
Rigid interactions, 101–103, 103–105
ROS. *See* Review of systems
Rosenham, D. L., 34, 41, 47
Roter, Deborah, 97

Roter Interaction Analysis Scale (RIAS),
    9, 97–100

Safety, 158
Satisfaction surveys, 30–31
Saturation, 96–97
Sayer, Jake, 6–7
Secret shopper patients, 32–33, 45–46.
    See also Unannounced standardized
    patients
SEGUE, 177
Self-selection bias, 31
Sharma, Gunjan, 43, 46, 62, 71
Simon's rule, 84, 99
Skepticism, 188–189
Skills and abilities, 17, 19, 89
Social courtesy, 115
Social security numbers, 43–44, 47–48
Social support, 17, 89
Soft skills, 121
SP. *See* Standardized patients
Spying, 66
Standardization, 106, 139
Standardized care, history of, 26–28
Standardized patients (SP), 32, 133–134.
    See also Unannounced standardized
    patients
Stemmler Medical Education Research
    Fund grants, 132
Stritch School of Medicine, 152
Subinternships, 125, 132–133
Surface acting, 177
Surveillance camera comparison, 161
Surveys, 30–31
Systems review approach to history
    taking, 105–109

Talmudic discussions, 84–85
Task focused biomedical information
    giving, 98
Teaching. *See also* Education
    of contextual reasoning, 123–131
    description of standard physician
        education in U.S. and, 121–123
    educators and, 194–196

gap between competence and
performance and, 134–136, 135t
overview of issue, 120
testing of, 131–134
Theory building approach to history
taking, 105–106, 109–112
To Err is Human (IOM), 28
Training. *See* Teaching
Translation, 142

Unannounced standardized
patients (USP)
advantages of use of, 60t
assessment of physicians studied
using, 96–97
detection of, 46–47
logistics of use of, 45–49
overview of, 31–39, 58–59, xviii
overview of study using, 39–45
results of study using, 49–53, 50t, 72, 73f
standardized patients vs.,
134–136, 135t
Underuse of medical resources, 54–56
Unions, 143–144, 145, 154, 159
United States Medical Licensing
Examination (USMLE), 122, 131
University of Illinois at Chicago (UIC),
29, 124–125, 131, 133, 152
USMLE. *See* United States Medical
Licensing Examination

USP. *See* Unannounced standardized
patients

VA. *See* Veterans Health Administration
Valuation of research, 144
Veering off topic, 100
Veterans Health Administration (VA)
continuous performance measurement
and feedback and, 141
electronic medical records system
of, 115
logistics of secret shopper patients
and, xviii
orders from to stop USP study, 47–49
real patients and, 59, 61–62
unannounced standardized patients
and, 39–45

Weaver, Fran, 48
Weingarten Rights, 159
"The Weird Sisters," 63
Wilson, Bette, 13–14
Workshop for teaching
contextualized care
gap between competence and
performance and, 134–136
limitations of, 135–136
overview of, 123–131
testing effectiveness of, 131–134

CPSIA information can be obtained
at www.ICGtesting.com
Printed in the USA
BVOW06s2104240117
474327BV00005BA/15/P